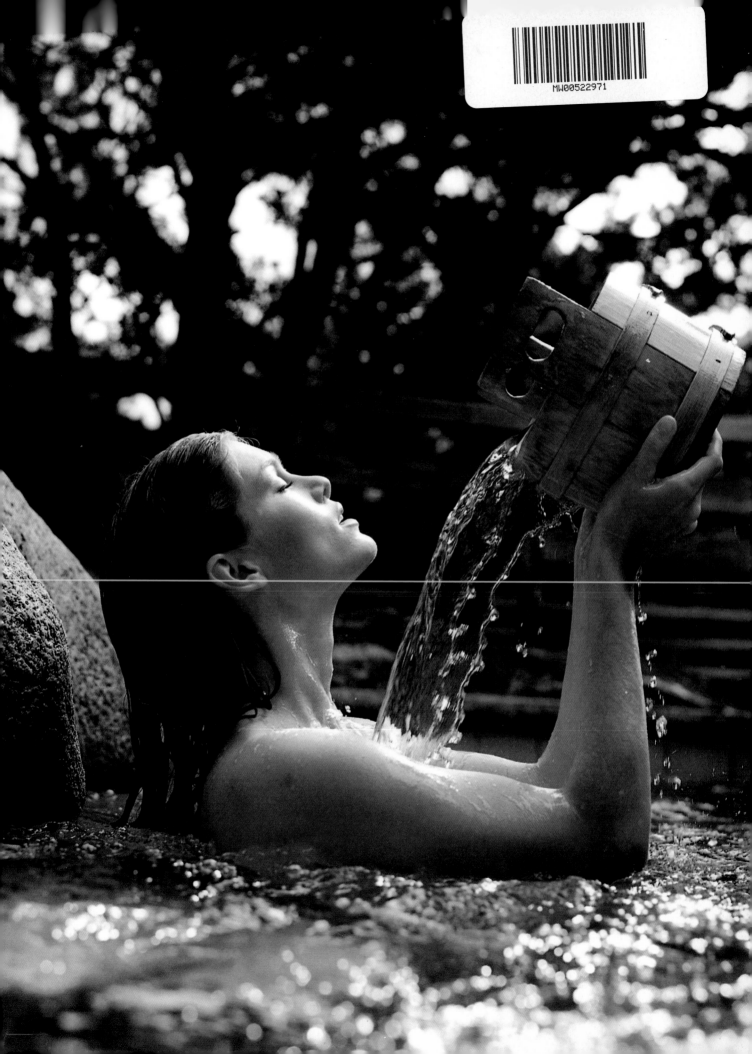

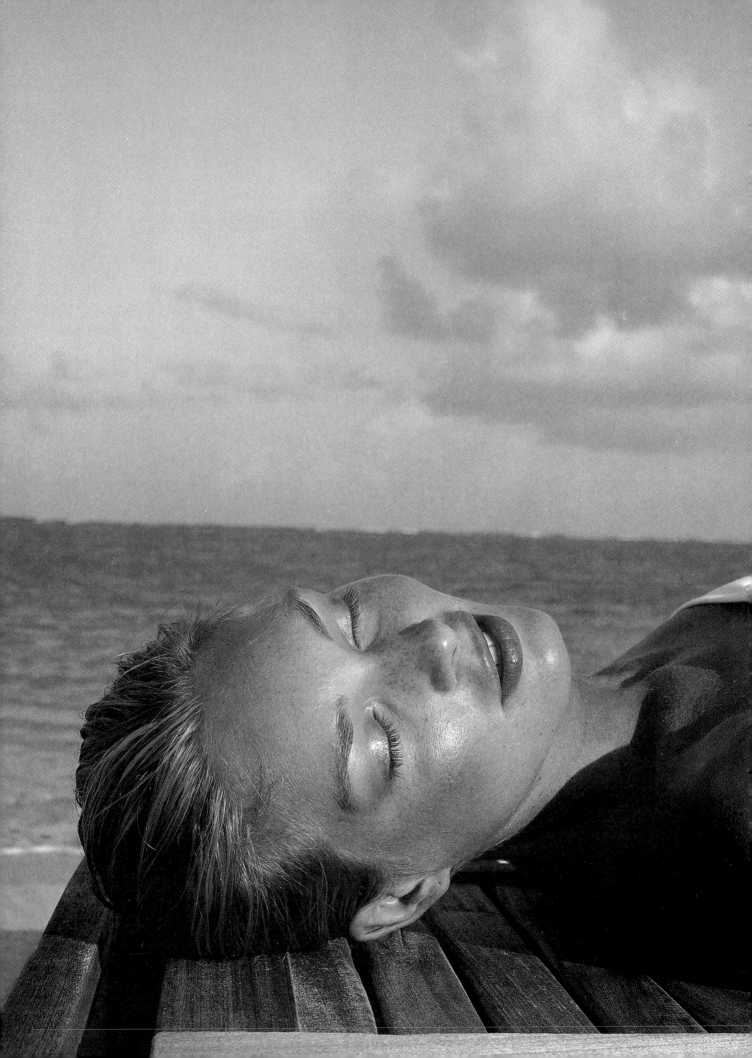

spa

PAMPER body and soul WITH

IDEAS FROM THE WORLD'S BEST SOURCES

KARENA CALLEN

EBURY PRESS
LONDON

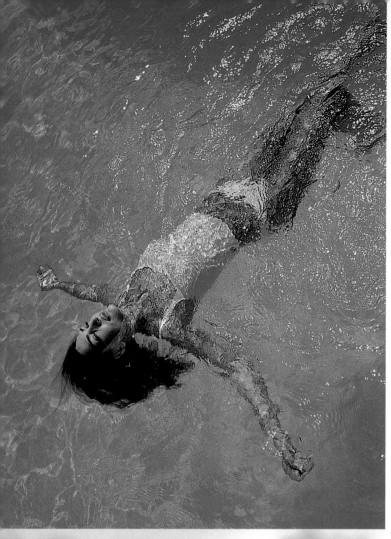

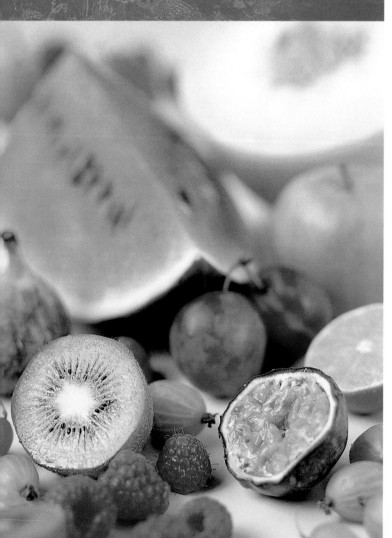

To my beautiful daughters, Shannon Emerald Georgia and Scarlet Alice Erin. Thank you for your love and for making me laugh.

First published in 2001

1 2 3 4 5 6 7 8 9 10

First published in the United Kingdom in 2001 by Ebury Press Random House, 20 Vauxhall Bridge Road, London SW1V 2SA

Random House Australia (Pty) Limited
20 Alfred Street, Milsons Point, Sydney,
New South Wales 2061, Australia

Random House New Zealand Limited
18 Poland Road, Glenfield, Auckland 10, New Zealand

Random House South Africa (Pty) Limited
Endulini, 5a Jubilee Road, Parktown 2193, South Africa

Random House UK Limited Reg. No. 954009

www.randomhouse.co.uk

A CIP catalogue record for this book is available from the British Library.

ISBN 0 09 187458 0

Editor: Emma Callery
Designer: Helen Lewis

Papers used by Ebury Press are natural, recyclable products made from wood grown in sustainable forests.

Printed and bound in Singapore by Tien Wah Press

CONTENTS

So near, so spa

Spa: a tiny word that has grown in significance. No longer merely associated with mineral springs and therapeutic taking-of-the-waters, Roman baths and Jane Austen, spa has taken on a new mantle that is hipper-than-hip. Be it in the form of to-die-for pampering products that line the shelves of the plushest beauty boutiques and most desirable department stores, mouth-watering and health-boosting cuisine or the ultimate in holiday destinations, you can't get away from the 's' word these days.

For me, and a growing number of spa-goers, spa is the ultimate chill-out mantra. Personally, I only have to think it, to repeat it silently a few times in my head, and my blood pressure drops, my heart rate halves and my muscles begin to soften and relax. It transports me back to my favourite spa resorts that I have been fortunate enough to visit during my 15 years as a pampered and privileged health and beauty director on glossy magazines.

And for millions of devotees, spa means time out from the hardships of life, the hubbub of urban living and the rigours of responsibility. Not only that, it is synonymous with peace, calm, tranquillity, me-time, space and getting-away-from-it-all. In fact, some fervent spa-worshippers are so devotional, that they have even gone as far as to suggest that 'spas are the new church'.

HAVE IT YOUR OWN WAY

But while escapism is an all-important part of the spa concept, in reality, few of us have the time or bank balance to allow us to pack up and check in every time we reach crisis point. Spa resorts may offer a once-in-a-while retreat from the madness, but ultimately, creating a sanctuary within our own space is the key to long-term stress survival. As a mother of three and with a decreasing amount of time to spend on myself, I no longer have the time or money to languor in the lap of luxury in faraway spa resorts. The closest I get these days to pampering is a candlelit soak in the tub, if I'm lucky. So I feel that I can speak from experience, as I've learned to make the most of a home-spa experience. And while my bathroom of the moment is a million miles away from my dream sanctuary, it's amazing what a soothing bath oil, a few scented tea lights and a pile of fluffy towels can do.

Indeed, it's perfectly possible to recreate the ambience that you might find at reknowned spas such as Canyon Ranch or Chiva-Som in your own bathroom by bringing in essential spa elements – aromas, accessories, indulgent pampering recipes for face and body, cosy, plump towels and sumptuous dressing gowns. They don't have to cost the earth.

It's this down-to-earth, practical philosophy that inspired this book. The tips, hints, recipes and inspiration gathered from deluxe and dreamy spas around the world allow you to sample the food, treatments and programmes that are on offer – and all within the comfort zone of your own home. Or, if you've picked this up following a spa stay, it's the perfect take-home treat that will inspire you to keep up the good work long after you've left the spa behind.

Karena Callen

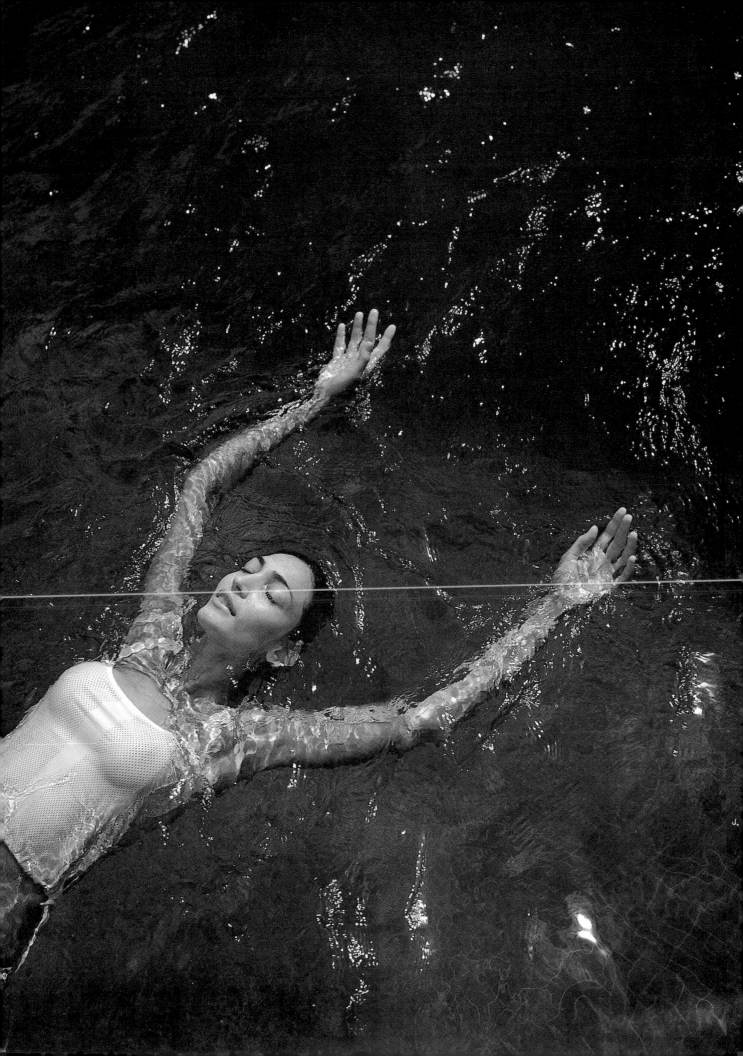

CREATING YOUR OWN
sanctuary

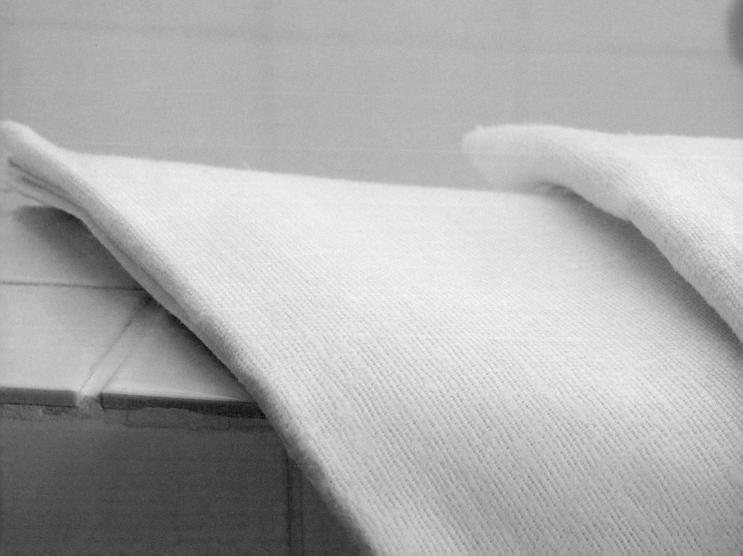

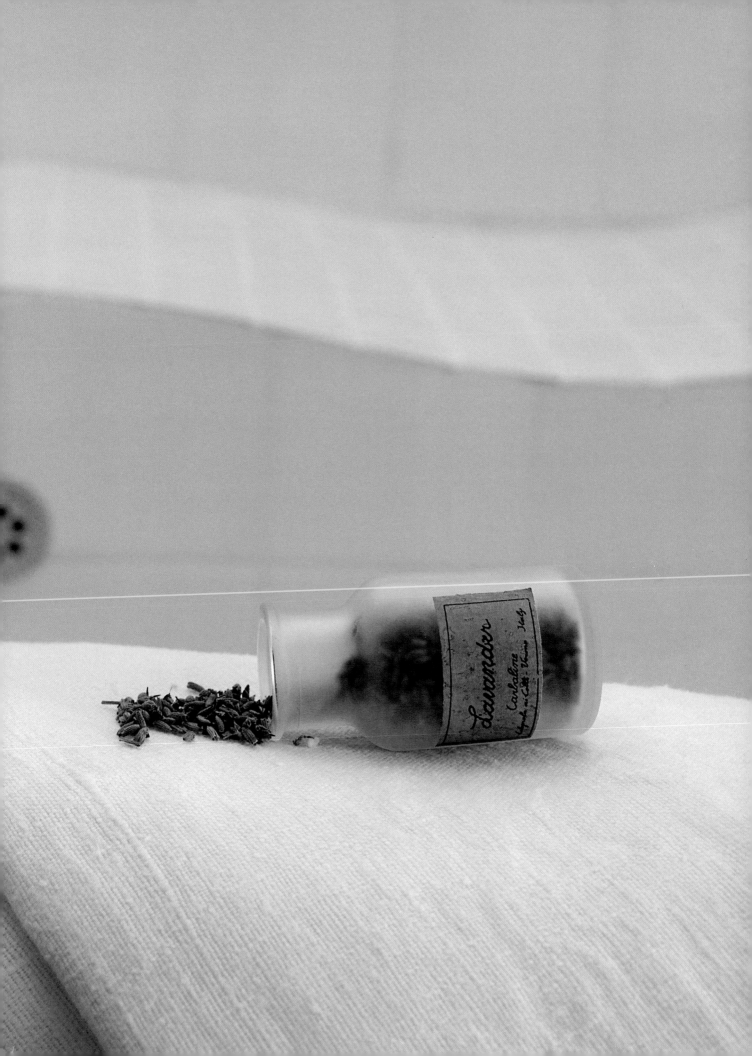

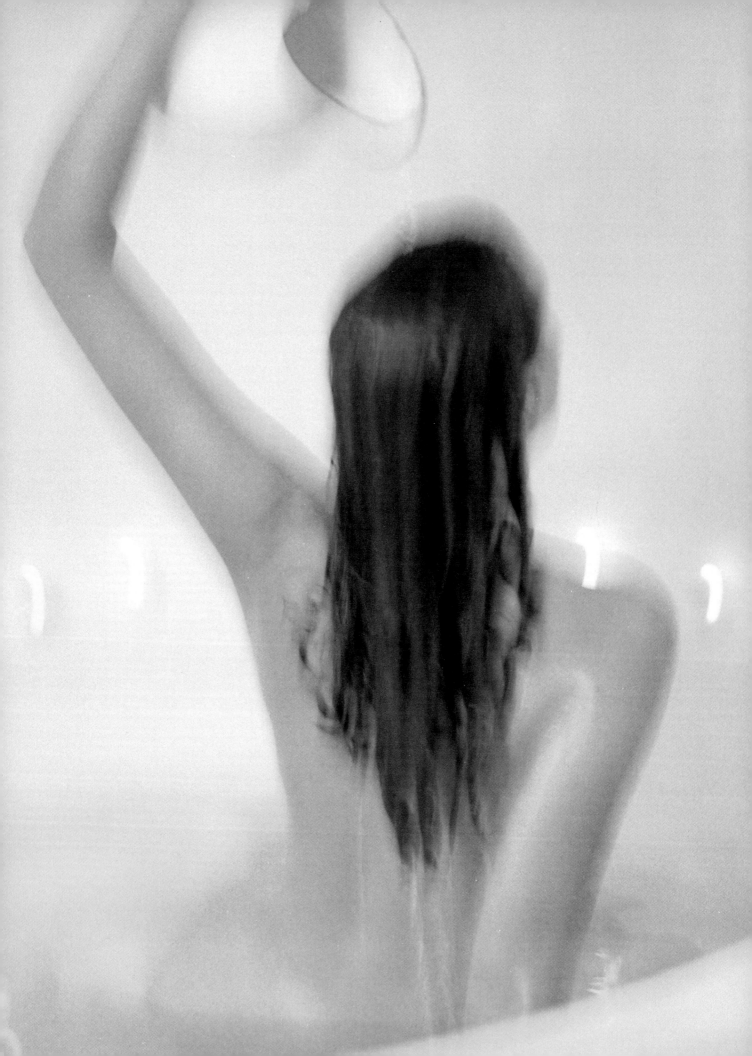

Comfort zone

We all need to retreat into our own private world from time to time, and – not surprisingly – most of us cite our bathroom as the ultimate chill out zone. Of course, there's a good reason for this. Water and bathing have long been associated with relaxation and well being. From our own primeval connection to water, to the fact that we all start out in a watery environment in the womb, you only have to look back at ancient cultures like the Egyptians, Greeks and Romans to see the importance of cleansing mind, body and spirit and communing with water. For many of us, the sensation of being in water, of bathing and showering, is a sensual one. And as a result, the bathroom, where water flows in abundance, tends to be one of our favourite comfort zones. It's the closest environment to a spa that we have access to at home, the place where we can cocoon ourselves, hide away from the outside world and get in touch with our most basic and natural needs. Not only that, but it is a realm where the majority of our senses can be pleasured. Textures, sounds and aromas are plentiful in a well-stocked, well-planned bathroom.

While going to a spa ensures the right environment for detoxifying and unwinding, for most of us, it's a once in a blue moon treat. Our own bathroom, however, is always close at hand. The good news is that you can create a taste of what you will find at a spa at home – and the best news is that it doesn't mean you have to call in the architects and a posse of builders and plumbers either. 'Small touches make all the difference,' says Lydia Sarfati, founder of the Beauty Company, Repechage. A pile of soft fluffy towels, a great wooden-handled body brush or some aromatic candles can take your plain old bathroom from dull to delicious in no time.

MINIMALIST DESIGN

Take a close look at the design of most spas and, no matter where they are in the world, one of the things you will notice is that they all tend to be uncluttered, pared-down and minimalist. Ornaments are carefully chosen and the number limited to keep distractions to a minimum. This Zen-like approach can be seen at spas as far removed geographically as the Golden Door on the west coast of North America and Chiva-Som in Thailand. Comfort comes from essentials like soothing aromatic oils in sleek, glass bottles and over-sized cuddly robes that swaddle naked skin.

In addition to vital prerequisites like towels, slippers and bathrobes, Sean Harrington, managing director of Elemis and creator of over 300 spas worldwide, cites lighting, music, stones and pebbles as favourite home spa elements. 'The perfect spa is a combination of elements that appeal to all the senses – music, lighting, textures, aromas – they all add up to create a harmonious environment.' Think about having dimmer switches fitted so that you can lower the lights for additional intimacy and cosiness and stock up on candles and nightlights. Lanterns and glass storm lights create soft, flickering light that is incredibly soothing and will help to put you into a state of deep relaxation. Aromas are also essential in creating your home spa retreat. Choose the aromas to suit your mood, whether you want to be calm, perk yourself up or encourage deep sleep.

Calming colour

The colours that you use in creating your sanctuary can go a long way to improving your mood and, according to colour therapists, can even help to stimulate your immune system and protect against illness. Using colour to uplift the spirits is hardly a new idea but one that more and more of us are absorbing into our everyday lives. Colour therapy is no longer the staple of alternative health practitioners – it has been readily adopted by everyone from beauty companies to interior designers.

WHITES

From the chalkiest of whites to creamier calico and canvas tones, white creates a feeling of space, light and purity, perfect for a spa-like environment. It will brighten dark spaces and spruce up and freshen a worn-out interior. White is a theme adopted at some of the most heavenly spa retreats. The Philippe Stark designed spas, Agua at Delano, Florida, USA and more recently at Agua at Sanderson, London, UK, have been created using celestial shades of white from the crispest brilliant white to the softest wax white. The result is a feeling of spaciousness, described by co-creator, Leila Fazel, as 'if you're floating on a cloud'. Paint walls, ceilings and woodwork with matt or eggshell paint in different hues of white. Give plain, sanded floorboards a new lease of life with white paint. Screen windows with billowing white muslin or white shutters.

BLUES

Being the colour of the water and the sky, blue always has a feel-good association. Used in many spas to create a sense of calm and relaxation, on a practical level, light translucent blues can also help to attract light into a dark room. From the palest of baby blues to more vibrant hyacinth or bluebell, blue brings with it a seaside, holiday feel and works well in the context of a bathroom. Deeper Moroccan-style cobalt and lapis blues can be teamed with mosaic wall tiles and terracotta floor tiles to create an exotic oasis.

GREENS

For a spa-style space, choose the palest, most light reflective greens and team them with fresh white, terracotta or sun-drenched yellow. On a spiritual note, green is the colour of the heart chakra. It is a famously soothing, harmonious colour that creates a natural environment. For a stronger statement, go for bolder shades such as turquoise and lime. Greens work well with natural wood or bamboo bathroom accessories and plain white baths and sinks. Recreate the tranquillity at Chiva-Som International Health Resort, Thailand, by using a combination of turquoise mosaic tiles, dark wooden accessories, pale green walls and potted palms and grasses.

VIOLET AND LAVENDER

Violet and lavender are often chosen because of their light attracting and purifying properties. In spiritual terms, violet is the colour of the 'third eye' – located in the centre of our brow – and is a truly sedative colour that helps to calm the central nervous system. Violet also helps us to tune in to our more intuitive side and therefore enables us to successfully access our higher consciousness.

Choose from the palest wash of lilac to stronger violets for a soothing, modern sanctuary. This spectrum of colours looks best with clean, simple accessories such as chrome, stainless steel, pale blonde wood and Perspex. Classic objects such as a fifties Arne Jacobsen butterfly chair look perfect against lilacs and lavenders.

YELLOWS

Like white, yellow helps open up a dingy, dark room and creates the illusion of space and light. Uplifting and awakening, sunny yellows always work as a mood enhancer and bring a sense of clarity and mental focus when used in room decoration. Incidentally, yellow relates to the solar plexus chakra, located just below the sternum.

Choose from creamy, buttery tones, vibrant egg yolk shades and deep mustards. Yellows and creams complement each other perfectly, creating a sunny, rustic feel. To complete the look, add simple pine or painted wood accessories, piles of soft, fluffy towels and canvas roman blinds or painted wooden shutters.

ORANGES

From the palest peach through to brilliant tangerine, the orange palette will warm up a cold space and make it feel cosier. Orange is the colour that represents the sacral chakra – just below the navel – the centre of pleasure and well being, so it's a very positive and creative shade to surround yourself with.

For a sensual sanctuary, combine it with terracotta tiles, simple earthenware containers and slatted wooden blinds for a feel that's similar to the Vista Clara Ranch Resort and Spa, New Mexico, USA. Or conjure up an environment reminiscent of the Nusa Dua Spa, Bali, Indonesia, by teaming orange with egg yolk yellow or dark green and adding dark wood or bamboo fixtures and fittings and simple glass bottles and jars filled with bath and body oils. Complete the mood by burning sandalwood or jasmine incense.

REDS

Red is not a relaxing colour, although darker shades can make a room feel cosy. Red represents the root chakra, located in the pelvic region, and is associated with passion, sexual energy and strength. If you do choose reds for your sanctuary stick to terracotta reds and deeper tones and steer clear of vivid or tomato reds. Shades of terracotta predominate at Rancho La Puerta, Baja California, Mexico. Teamed with other vibrant shades like strong, deep pink, egg yolk yellow and cobalt blue and natural materials like stripped wood, you can create a Rancho feel in your own sanctuary. Look out for Mexican-style pottery and tiles to complete the look.

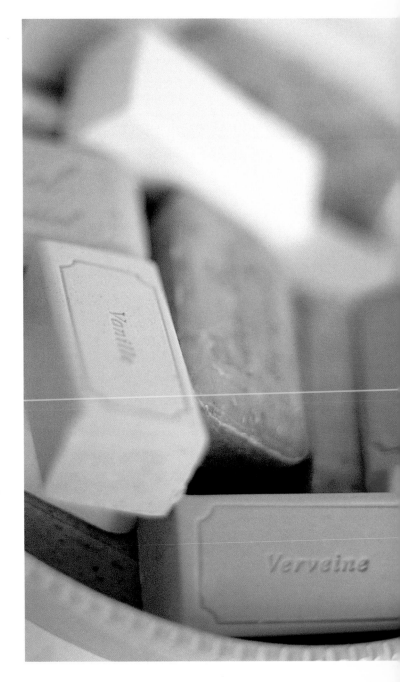

Aromas

Scent has the power to transport us not only to other times in our lives, but to faraway places, destinations that we may have visited in reality or merely in our dreams. Each spa that I have visited has its own distinctive aroma that when smelt even years after, takes me back to my time spent there. In particular, Ten Thousand Waves, Santa Fe, New Mexico, emits the most wonderful mix of cedar and sage, native to that part of the state – one sniff of either and I am floating in a hot tub under the stars. Burning oils or incense in your bathroom will help you to create your own little temple, a space that is sacred to you and to your family. This might be just the opportunity you need to remind yourself of a favourite spa or vacation, in which case, choose a scent that conjures images of that place.

LAVENDER

Always reminiscent of Provence, lavender is a clean, fresh scent that has potent relaxing properties. Hang bunches of dried lavender in linen cupboards to scent your towels and laundry or burn lavender essential oil or scented candles in your bathroom to create a wonderful summer breeze through the room.

YLANG YLANG

One of the most popular essential oils used in tropical spas such as the Nusa Dua Spa, Bali, Indonesia, ylang ylang is renowned for its anti-depressant properties not to mention the fact that it is a powerful aphrodisiac. Ylang ylang combines well with woody aromas such as vetiver and sensual oils like jasmine and rose.

JASMINE

Used in profusion in Southeast Asian spas, jasmine has incredibly uplifting euphoric and sensual properties. Add a few drops of jasmine oil to your bath, burn it in an oil burner or, if you can track one down, bathe by the light of a jasmine scented candle. Sheer bliss.

PATCHOULI

For some, patchouli brings back too many memories of the hippy trail, but for others it is one of the most arousing, sexy fragrances. Popular in many of the Malaysian and Balinese spas, it is used not only as a perfume and room scent but to treat skin conditions as diverse as eczema and acne. Use in small doses or you could find your loved ones leaving home. Patchouli incense creates the most wonderful earthy aroma conducive to a meditative state.

SAGE

One of my favourite aromas at home, sage is a real cleanser. Used in many Native American Indian ceremonies, it is often used in the form of smudge sticks – tightly bound bundles of sage – that are set alight and then snuffed out and the smoke used to rid a room of any bad vibes. If you like the smell of sage, grow some fresh in terracotta pots and keep that in your bathroom. Otherwise, you can find sage-based room fragrances, oils and incense if you hunt around.

SANDALWOOD

Inhaling sandalwood is like stepping in to the souk in Marrakech or a Southeast Asian spa.

Sandalwood has been used for centuries in purification rituals and is said to have potent mind and body relaxing properties. Sandalwood oil is used at many of the Asian spas, particularly in massage, and is also very good for re-balancing oily skin (see the facial blends given on page 100). Burn the essential oil or buy it in incense form for a traditional sandalwood experience.

EUCALYPTUS

A favourite with Australian spas, eucalyptus has a wonderful medicinal aroma that really clears sinuses and helps to fight off colds and flu. Team this particular oil with tea tree oil for a really traditional Antipodean rescue remedy. Eucalyptus works very well in the shower too. Put a few drops on to a sponge and then vigorously massage it into your skin as you shower.

TEA TREE

Another favourite with Australian spas, tea tree has powerful antiseptic properties and is a great room purifier. Mix it with a little peppermint, eucalyptus and lavender for a deep-cleansing effect. Add a few drops to a vaporiser or bowl of warm water.

CEDARWOOD

Popular at southwestern spas in the USA, cedarwood is excellent for boosting flagging energy levels and low self-esteem. It works well in combination with sandalwood, ylang ylang, sage and jasmine. Put a few drops in an oil burner or on a damp cotton wool ball placed behind a radiator for a woody, outdoorsy aroma.

SCENTING YOUR SANCTUARY

Create different moods by hand-blending your own essential oil combinations.

Purification: if you are in need of a detox, try this blend of cleansing oils. Add 2 drops of tea tree oil to 3 drops of eucalyptus and 2 drops of peppermint. Put into an oil burner or vaporiser to purify your sanctuary. This blend is also perfect for chasing away colds and 'flu. Tea tree is an excellent antiseptic, while eucalyptus helps to clear the nasal passages and peppermint can help to reduce a temperature.

Sacred space: when you need to retreat and cocoon yourself, blend 3 drops of lavender with 2 drops of sage and 2 drops of frankincense, add to 1 tablespoon of a carrier oil, such as aloe vera or avocado oil, and add to a warm bath just as you step into it. The aroma will fill the room too, leaving you feeling cosy and nurtured.

Chill out: burning the candle at both ends? Living life in the fast lane and can't put on the brakes? Surround yourself with this blend to bring you back to a slower, steadier pace. Add 5 drops of lavender to 4 drops of patchouli, 3 drops of rose and 3 drops of chamomile. Add to an oil burner to scent the room or to a bowl of steaming water and inhale for a few minutes. To make your own room scent, add a few drops of each oil to an atomiser containing distilled water and spray in the room, on to your bathrobe and on to your pillow at night.

Laughter: when life is getting you down, use this uplifting blend to boost your spirits. Combine 4 drops of rose with 4 drops of tangerine, 2 drops of geranium and 2 drops of bergamot and add to an oil burner or a small bowl of warm water placed on or near a radiator. Let the aroma surround you to bring back your sense of humour.

Fixtures and fittings

If you take a close look at the design of most spas, no matter where they are in the world, one of the things they all have in common is that they tend to be uncluttered, pared-down and often minimalist. Comfort comes from sensual elements like aromatic oils in sleek glass bottles, over-sized cuddly robes, flickering candles and incense burners and dreamily soft slippers. 'Comfort is crucial,' says international spa creator and managing director of beauty company E'Spa, Susan Harmsworth. 'Investing in simple but luxurious accessories and storage containers to keep things ordered ensures that your space looks crisp and clean so you won't have to spend your valuable relaxation time having to move things around or rummaging for that favourite body cream.'

SIMPLE STORAGE

There is a huge difference between a spa and a home, but in terms of achieving a spa look, tidying away clutter is key. Keep an eye out for elegant glass jars in which to keep essential prerequisites like cotton buds and cotton wool. Stainless steel or metallic canisters look orderly and give a modern feel on a plain wooden shelf or window sill, while hand-made Shaker wooden boxes offer a more rustic option, especially when teamed with generous wicker laundry baskets.

When it comes to cupboards, search antique shops and flea markets for old-style larders that can be painted with eggshell paint to match walls and woodwork. Hotel-style chrome trolleys are both stylish and ergonomic, as they can be easily moved around when stocked with bathing essentials and piles of soft, fluffy towels and flannels.

TOWEL RAILS

Whether you choose sleek chrome hotel-style towel rails or simple New Mexican inspired wooden towel ladders, a place to hang your towels close to the bath is a real essential. Heated towel rails are particularly worth investing in, especially for winter, when there really is nothing so appealing as wrapping your body in a swathe of plush, warm towelling.

Alternatively, you can prop a simple wooden rail against the wall over an existing radiator to ensure that your towels and bathrobe are warmed up. Or consider painting up a wooden clothes airer to do a similar job.

BEAUTIFUL BATHS

From luxurious break-the-bank Japanese-style wooden tubs hewn out of aromatic cedar to cast iron junk yard finds, the perfect bath depends entirely on your own taste. Given the choice, I'd go for a free-standing, Victorian-style cast iron tub any day. I love the vast, deep space and the fact that I can have a pile of books at one side and a table with scented candles and a battery-operated CD player and radio for essential soothing music on the other.

Whichever bath you choose, make sure you invest in a decent plumbing and water heating system to ensure that you have a constant, copious supply of hot water. There's nothing worse than having to wait hours for your bath to run or finding that you have three drops of hot water when you are craving a luxurious soak. The initial expense may be greater, but if it makes for longer-term relaxation it has to be worth it.

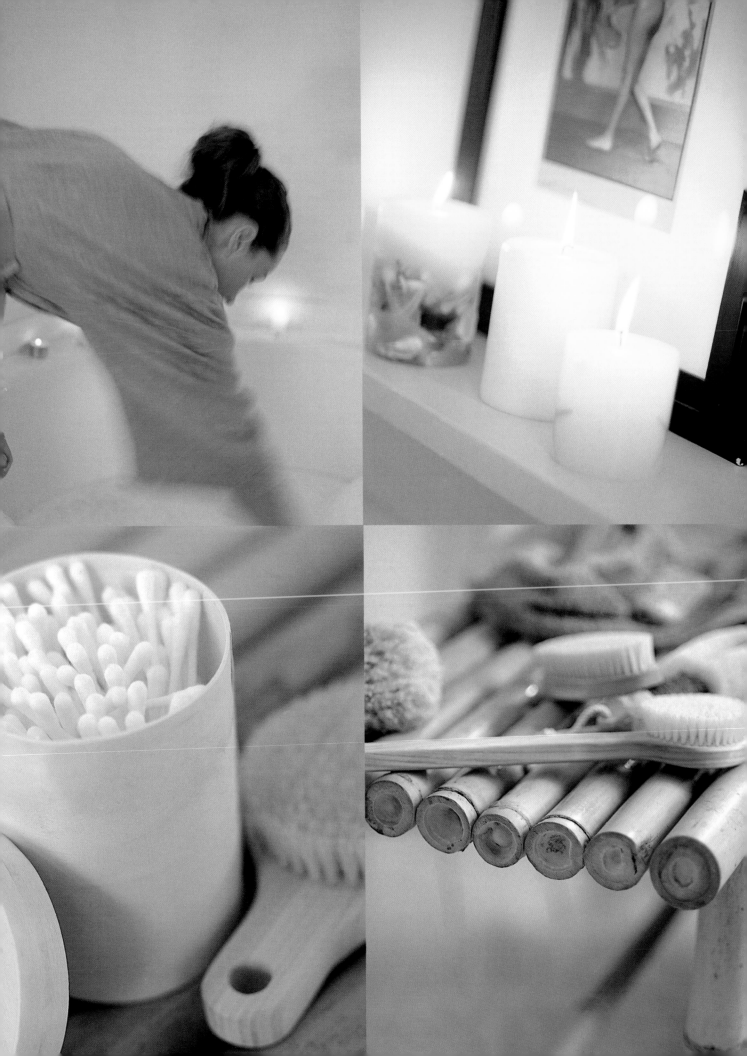

POWER SHOWERS

There's nothing more invigorating than starting the day under a stream of gorgeous, skin cleansing water, delivered at high pressure from an efficient shower. If you live in an area where the water pressure is low, a power shower is by far the best option, unless you want to find yourself standing under a feeble trickle of water that alternates hot and cold. If you enjoy a real soak, look out for a shower with a large, chrome head, almost like an enormous watering can, which delivers a wonderful waterfall cascade. For those who prefer high-pressure needle-like jets, compact American-style six-prong showerheads are the best option.

MATERIAL CHOICES

• Toughened glass sinks with chrome fittings will enhance any modern, minimalist sanctuary.
• Stainless steel is both functional and streamline, although it may need to be treated with extra care to avoid scratching. Can look a little clinical, but works well with crisp white woodwork and softer touches like blonde wooden accessories.
• Ceramic sinks can be found in a variety of shapes and sizes from square Belfast-style basins to modern, sculpted sinks. Easy to keep clean, they always look pure and pristine.
• Natural and reconstructed marble basins work in synch with dark Japanese-style woods such as mahogany and teak and simple, streamlined accessories. Reconstructed marble basins are made by combining powdered marble and resin and tend to be harder wearing than natural marble.

SPA AND WHIRLPOOL BATHS

If you have the opportunity and the budget to have a complete bathroom makeover, putting in a spa or whirlpool bath will make even more of the time spent in your private sanctuary. Choose from spa baths that pump warm air into the bath water, whirlpool baths that re-circulate the water or whirlpool spas that circulate a combination of water and air.

Choose from large hot-tub-style circular baths to more traditional roll-top shapes and ensure that you have space for the pump, which needs to be installed either directly under the bath or in a storage cupboard. Spa baths do need to be installed by an expert and you will need to check that all electrical components are protected by a circuit breaker.

BASINS AND SINKS

Whether you opt for a basic porcelain sink or a high tech stainless steel basin, ensure that you invest in one that suits your everyday needs. In addition to being an artefact, your basin should be practical – deep enough to allow you to dunk your hands and face if you need to and to ensure that you don't end up with a waterlogged floor. Take your pick from pedestal, wall-hung or countertop styles, depending on the look you're after. In terms of materials, again the world's your oyster (see left).

Taps are also important – they need to be functional, not just decorative. Again, it's a matter of choice what style you pick and the variety is truly awe inspiring. Choose from traditional pillar-style taps, basin mixer or single lever monobloc taps. Putting new taps on an old sink can smarten it up instantly.

Step into the light

Lighting is crucial in helping to create the right atmosphere in your sanctuary. From downlighters to candles, task lighting to spotlights, choosing the kind of illumination you want depends entirely on personal taste and individual needs. Brilliant, blazing light is not an essential in a bathroom sanctuary. In fact, many types of artificial lighting can be cold and unflattering, so make the most of natural light during the day by choosing a colour scheme that is light reflective and ensuring that window coverings are as translucent as possible. I don't care what any design gurus say about the modernity of fluorescent lighting – it's incredibly cold and unforgiving. If you want to create a really intimate soothing environment, it is best avoided altogether.

NATURAL LIGHT
Having a bathroom with windows and natural light will make life a whole lot easier. You can manipulate the light coming in by your choice of window treatments. Shutters and Venetian blinds allow privacy while letting daylight filter through. Opaque glass or transparent gauzy curtains again give an element of privacy while allowing light to come through.

AMBIENT LIGHT
Nothing creates a more soothing, relaxing atmosphere than candlelight. For the ultimate in relaxing bath-time pampering, candlelight is hard to beat. Invest in a dozen or so little tea lights or dinner lights in glass containers and place them around your bath or on shelves around the room,

ensuring they are not near anything that's flammable. Large pillar candles also throw a beautiful light that's perfect for bathing by.

OVERALL LIGHTING
By far the most pleasing form of overall lighting, halogen downlighters cast an even, pure light over a room and can be dimmed for a softer effect and combined with candlelight in the evening. In addition, because they can be recessed into the ceiling, they don't intrude decoratively. Perfect for creating a modern, minimalist haven.

TASK LIGHTING
Spotlights and mirror lights provide a clear, direct light source and are a necessity, particularly if you are performing grooming acts such as eyebrow tweezing or applying make-up. Have them put on a separate switch to your main bathroom lighting so that they can be turned on only when you need their services.

TIPS
• While aesthetics are obviously key when picking bathroom lighting, safety is paramount. Ensure that the lights you choose are suitable for bathroom use before fitting them. And for extra security, use a qualified electrician.
• Ceiling lights should be sealed within a plastic steam or waterproof diffuser.
• Avoid fitting wall-mounted light switches within your bathroom and opt instead for pull-cord fittings. Better still, place light switches outside the room.

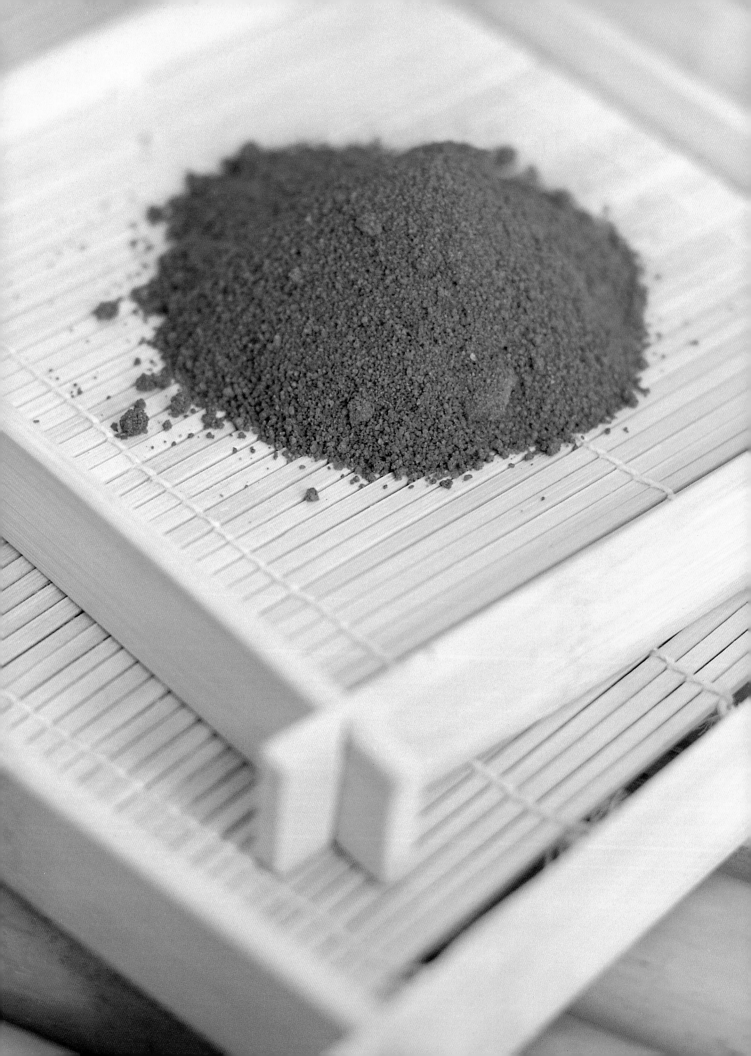

Textures

While the appearance and aroma of your sanctuary are crucial in creating a haven that's your own, never forget that the sense of touch is of the utmost importance. The feel of the objects that you choose for your bathroom can improve the quality of your time spent luxuriating. Textures can be complementary – the warmth of a wooden floor, piles of huge, fluffy bath sheets, rounded weathered glass storage jars and bottles – or you can choose to put opposites together for an equally pleasing sensation. Cool, smooth limestone flooring teamed with a soft, looped towelling bath mat or a weathered wooden duckboard work beautifully together. Billowy muslin curtains, teamed with plain white-washed plaster walls and piles of hand-picked pebbles from beach-combing trips please not only your eyes, but your hands, as you explore the different textures while in your sanctuary.

ROUGH AND READY

Roughness is not a texture that might immediately spring to mind in association with a sanctuary. On the contrary, many natural materials – think pumice, sisal, coir – are conducive to a peaceful, calming environment and are often irregular and rough to the touch. The trick is to combine the rough with the smooth to create a rounded, textural experience that combines as many pleasurable sensations as possible. Roughly hewn stone jars and shallow bowls are perfect storage containers for bath salts, piles of scented, hand-made soaps and collections of shells and driftwood. A sisal mat or runner feels stimulating under foot after a long soak in the tub. You can also transform a bland or featureless room by adding salvaged tongue-and-groove panelling or by choosing weather-beaten accessories, such as a distressed painted wooden chair or cupboard.

SMOOTH

Rounded objects and smooth surfaces beg to be caressed and enjoyed. Especially suited to the bathroom, smooth textures – from polished limestone flooring to a marble fireplace, piles of sandblasted cobbles and gently curved glass jars and bottles – are a pleasure to hold and touch. Spherical objects, like marbles and pebbles, look beautiful displayed in glass jars or in smooth, shallow bowls and can be used as meditation tools. Simply roll two large marbles or rounded pebbles between your fingers or in your palm as you relax in a warm bath. Close your eyes and focus on the rolling action to soothe away stress. Heap bars of smooth, aromatic soaps into bowls and jars to add colour and texture.

Smooth floors, like limestone and marble, also feel and look clean in a bathroom – but be aware that they can be slippery when wet. Keep a wooden duckboard or absorbent bath mat to hand for post-bath safety.

SOFT

Nothing compares to the luxurious sensation of being swathed in a soft, thick-piled towel or robe after bathing. It takes us back to our childhood, makes us feel warm and secure and on a practical note, dries us quickly. Stockpile jumbo-sized bath sheets, robes and towelling bath slippers and store them in an airing cupboard for extra comfort. Replace your towels on a regular basis – old towels tend to become threadbare and lose their softness. Seek out the plushest, velour towels that are ideal for children, as they tend to have a more velvety texture than traditional looped towelling. Keep a plentiful supply of skin softening and soothing body oils, creams and lotions for post-bath massage – nothing feels more relaxing than a rub down.

Accessories

To make the most of your home spa, stock up on versatile accessories that not only look beautiful decoratively, but that enhance skin, mood and your immediate environment. Fill a shallow wooden bowl with natural sponges or piles of multi-coloured hand-made soaps; hang body brushes on a simple Shaker-style peg rail and stockpile fine muslin cloths and flannels in a wire-fronted bathroom cupboard for easy access.

SPONGES

Skin has more affinity with natural sponges than with synthetic ones. Use them with soap or a favourite bath foam to achieve a sensual lather. A tip to prolong the life of a natural sponge is to soak it in vinegar once in a while. This will literally pickle and preserve it. Always make sure you rinse it well after bathing or showering and place it somewhere warm to dry.

BODY BRUSHES

Sisal and bristle body brushes can be hung up on hooks and peg rails, being both practical and ornamental. Body brushing is highly recommended by many therapists to stimulate the body's lymphatic system – basically a kind of waste disposal. When stressed or under par, the lymphatic system can become sluggish, and a daily session of skin brushing where you brush lightly across dry skin, always working towards the heart, is thought to be beneficial.

LOOFAHS

Brilliant for scrubbing parts that are tricky to reach, fibrous loofahs help to stimulate the circulation, exfoliate the skin and generally work a bit like a natural steel wool pad. They need to be well rinsed and dried in order to preserve them.

MUSLIN CLOTHS AND FLANNELS

Best for cleansing sensitive skin, muslin cloths and cotton flannels exfoliate gently and when combined with a cleansing oil or cream, they are super effective skin polishers. If the skin on your face is playing up and misbehaving, soak a muslin cloth in very hot water to which you should add a few drops of tea tree and lavender essential oils and then place over your face as you relax in a warm bath.

PUMICE STONES

With its neutral colour and organic texture, pumice stone blends in equally well with a very modern or rustic-style sanctuary. Ideal for polishing away hard skin on feet, especially heels, pumice comes in a variety of shapes and sizes.

BATH AND SEA SALTS

Fill glass apothecary and flip-top preserve jars with all kinds of sea and bath salts. Not only are they perfect for creating instant skin-softening body scrubs when mixed with a little oil, they add colour and texture to the bathroom environment.

PEBBLES AND COBBLES

Beach-combed pebbles and cobbles not only look beautiful piled on shelves and on the floor – they can be used for massage too. Warm them in hot water with a little oil and use them to massage hands and feet while soaking in the bath.

CHILL-OUT MUSIC

Music is one of the most powerful mediums that you can use to transport you from the real world to your own personal Nirvana. Tune in to those sounds that will help you to release tension, bottled-up emotions and, in some cases, allow you to access a higher level of consciousness.

Divine Bliss

by Shri Anandi Ma (Sounds True)
Blissful Indian devotional music that will help you to achieve your own trance-like state. Perfect to meditate to.

Gone to Earth

by David Sylvian (Virgin Records)
Deeply soothing songs to take you to another world that's far from the stressful one you currently inhabit. One to listen to while you wallow in the bath.

The Moon and the Melodies

by Harold Budd, Simon Raymonde, Robin Guthrie and Elizabeth Fraser (4AD)
Be prepared to be lulled and tranquillised by tantalising vocals and wonderful ethereal melodies. The perfect soothe-you-to-sleep sounds.

Spirit Horses: The Music of James DeMars

by R. Carlos Nakai (Canyon)
Eerie and beautiful, this Native American flute music, as recommended by Westward Look Resort, Arizona, USA, will carry you to another plain of consciousness. The ideal accompaniment to yoga or meditation.

Big Calm

by Morcheeba (Indochina Records)
Modern chill-out music at its best – and not a twee, twangy sound or dolphin click in evidence. If you hate the grating New Age music passed off as relaxing, you'll love this. Soak in the tub, relax with a face mask or just curl up on your beanbag.

Symphonies 40 & 38

by Mozart, performed by the English Chamber Orchestra (Decca)
Guaranteed to uplift your mood and divert your attention from the hassles of everyday life.

Southern Exposure

by Alex de Grassi (Windham Hill Records)
Gorgeous solo guitar that takes you to sun-filled landscapes and big skies with billowing clouds.

The Pearl

by Harold Budd and Brian Eno (EG Records)
Unlock pent-up tension by playing this deliciously composed ambient treasury. Better than any lullaby, put it on and you'll be soothed into a state of total tranquillity.

Astral Weeks

by Van Morrison (Warner Brothers)
Stunningly beautiful lyrics and melodies paint dreamy pictures that will leave you feeling completely 'at one' with the universe.

Arabesque

A compilation by Momo (Gut Records)
Guaranteed to chase away the blues, this up-tempo, North African chill-out music will make you smile rather than sleep. Put this on after a hard day at the office and you'll find yourself transported to exotic locations without having to leave the cosiness of your own sanctuary.

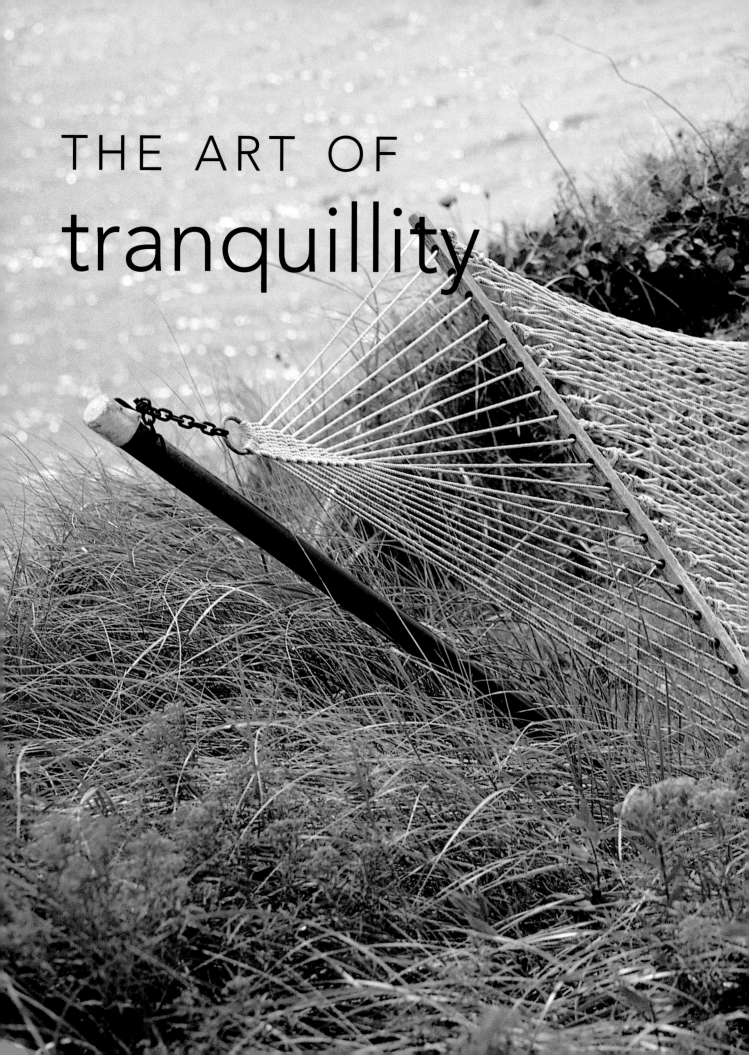

THE ART OF
tranquillity

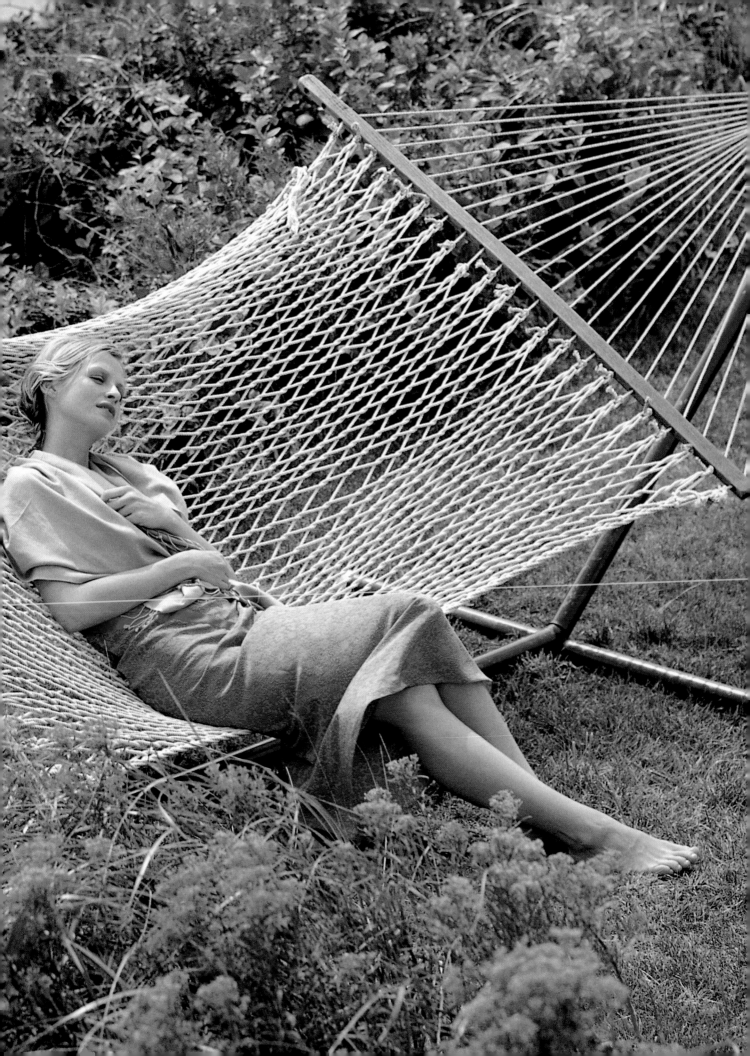

Learn to relax

If I ever do have the chance to book a spa vacation, my motivation could be summed up by the desperate need for one thing – relaxation. Peace, calm, tranquillity – call it what you will, there is just not enough of this precious attribute in our modern, stress-filled lives. We are all guilty of doing too much, biting off more than we can chew and running on empty. But all too often we are so busy running to stand still, that we do not stop to think of the consequences. Burn-out, fatigue, stress-related illness and insomnia are all the result of overload.

THE STRESS FACTOR
Of course, we all need an element of stress in our lives in order to function, otherwise we would probably just curl up on the sofa and refuse to move. Deadlines, financial pressures, the demands of family, friends and children all motivate us in both a positive and negative way. We all get wrapped up in our own stress cycles and become so accustomed to the physical and emotional demands that stress puts on us, that we become accustomed to living under stress. In physical terms, this eventually takes its toll. The reason? When we are under stress, be it stuck in a traffic jam or in a job interview, our bodies undergo physiological changes. Adrenaline races through our veins, raising our cortisol levels – one of the main stress hormones. As a result, our energy levels soar – in primitive times this fight or flight response fuelled our ability to defend ourselves from predators or, if we saw fit, to run away super fast. But just as energy levels rise and our heart beats rapidly, we fall into a vicious circle of highs and lows. Eventually, our adrenal glands can become fatigued, and thyroxin – a hormone that controls our metabolism – becomes depleted, leaving us feeling exhausted and without any *joie de vivre*. An all-too-familiar scenario for a growing number of us.

THE ANTI-STRESS SPA SOLUTION
Enough gloom. There is a simple solution to this modern dilemma, and that is to follow the pathway that the ancient cultures laid down in order to keep life in balance and to stay free of disease. That is, to learn the art of tranquillity, to relax, to do nothing, to chill out or to contemplate – basically, to return our minds and bodies to a Zen-like state. This may be easier said than done, yet it is not as difficult or monumental as you might think. The secret is to take up a specific technique that allows you to unwind. Transcendental meditation is my own particular key whereas for others more active methods such as t'ai chi, yoga or aikido will do the trick. It's all down to finding out what suits your physical and emotional needs and this is often a case of trial and error.

Relaxation techniques are a growing part of spa culture with practices like yoga and t'ai chi becoming more and more of a draw to spa goers. With this in mind, I've asked the experts at leading spas around the world to devise simple programmes that you can do at home, based on the extensive menus on offer at their particular resorts. Take the time to road test the techniques for yourself. Once you find the method that's right for you, all it takes is regular practice and the results can be far reaching.

INSTANT STRESS-BUSTER TIPS

At work, meeting deadlines or dealing with a difficult person, taking a deep breath and counting to ten could quite literally be what you need. During times of overload cultivate the art of stepping back to look at the 'larger picture'. To release stress from any situation, distance yourself mentally for a few minutes. Here, stress management expert, Phyllis Pilgrim, based at Rancho La Puerta, Baja California, Mexico, shares her quick-fix ways to help release the stress in your life.

1 Move physically out of the situation – go to a different room or go outside into the fresh air.
2 Inhale, stretching your arms up, then exhale and lower your arms. Repeat 5-10 times.
3 Take in a deep breath and count to ten as you exhale. With the exhalation, let problems and difficulties go.
4 Inhale positivity and solutions to your problems. Repeat 10 times.
5 Lower your shoulders and exhale. Roll your shoulders forward, then back. Repeat 10 times.
6 Smile as you inhale.
7 Exhale with strong exhalation sounds, blowing out your difficulties.
8 Breathe freely and stretch in any way you like.
9 Invite spaciousness and freedom into your consciousness.

An ancient Chinese exercise called ki can also physically help you to distance yourself psychologically from the immediate problem at hand and allow yourself the ability to rediscover the larger perspective.

1 Stand with your feet slightly apart, knees bent and hands over abdomen.
2 Breathe rhythmically and attune to your own energy (ki) through your breath.
3 Breathe in and lift your arms slowly to shoulder level – assess the situation.
4 As you exhale, step back with your right foot, bring your hands to your chest, elbows out sideways. Look at the larger picture.
5 Inhale, turn palms out then exhale and sweep arms forward and sideways – clear away the clutter.
6 Inhale, bringing hands in sideways to shoulders, palms out. Exhale, pressing hands out sideways – create the space you are comfortable working in.
7 Inhale, stepping back, foot forward again, lowering arms down to the side and up the front of your body – stepping back into the situation, seeing it from your new perspective.
8 Exhale, pressing palms down to position hands in front of abdomen – return to the situation, calm and peaceful.
9 Repeat, placing the left foot back.

INSTANT CALMERS

There will be days when stress levels are soaring but you just can't squeeze in a calming session of yoga or meditation. The solution? Try one of these stress-reducing remedies.

Herbal helpers: there are a number of tried and tested herbal remedies that help your body to cope with stress more effectively and, in turn, will make you feel less harassed.

• Kava kava can be taken in supplement, infusion or tincture form and will give you an instant shot of calm.

• Panax ginseng helps the body to adapt to long-term stress but needs to be taken over a long period of time in order to be effective. Take in tincture or supplement form.

• Valerian root works well for those suffering from nervous tension and insomnia. Make an infusion of the root and take 250 ml up to three times a day.

• Chamomile and cowslip are also effective relaxants. Make an infusion with the petals and drink 250 ml two or three times a day.

Aromatherapy assets: specific essential oils extracted from flowers and plants can help to reduce the symptoms of stress overload and promote relaxation. Add them to your bath water or to a carrier oil and use to massage your temples, wrists and hands for instant at-your-desk relief.

• *For tranquillity:* mix 2 drops petitgrain, 3 drops vetiver and 3 drops clary sage.

• *For meditation:* mix 2 drops cedarwood, 2 drops sandalwood, 2 drops frankincense and 2 drops rose.

• *To soothe:* mix 3 drops chamomile, 2 drops mandarin and 2 drops ylang ylang.

• *To unwind:* mix 2 drops geranium, 2 drops lavender and 2 drops myrrh.

Flower power: flower remedies, such as those created by Dr Edward Bach and more recent versions like the Australian Bush Flower Essences, work on the emotions. Try these blends in your bath water when you are feeling worn to a frazzle.

• *To help overcome an office crisis:* mix 2 drops each of white chestnut, walnut, vervain, olive, rock water, mustard, oak and gentian.

• *To help prevent sleepless nights:* mix 2 drops each of olive, rock rose, white chestnut, impatiens and vervain.

• *When you are feeling down in the dumps:* mix 2 drops each of gentian, walnut, gorse, wild rose, sweet chestnut and willow.

• *When you are burnt out:* mix 2 drops each of wild rose, walnut, mustard, oak, olive, elm and gorse.

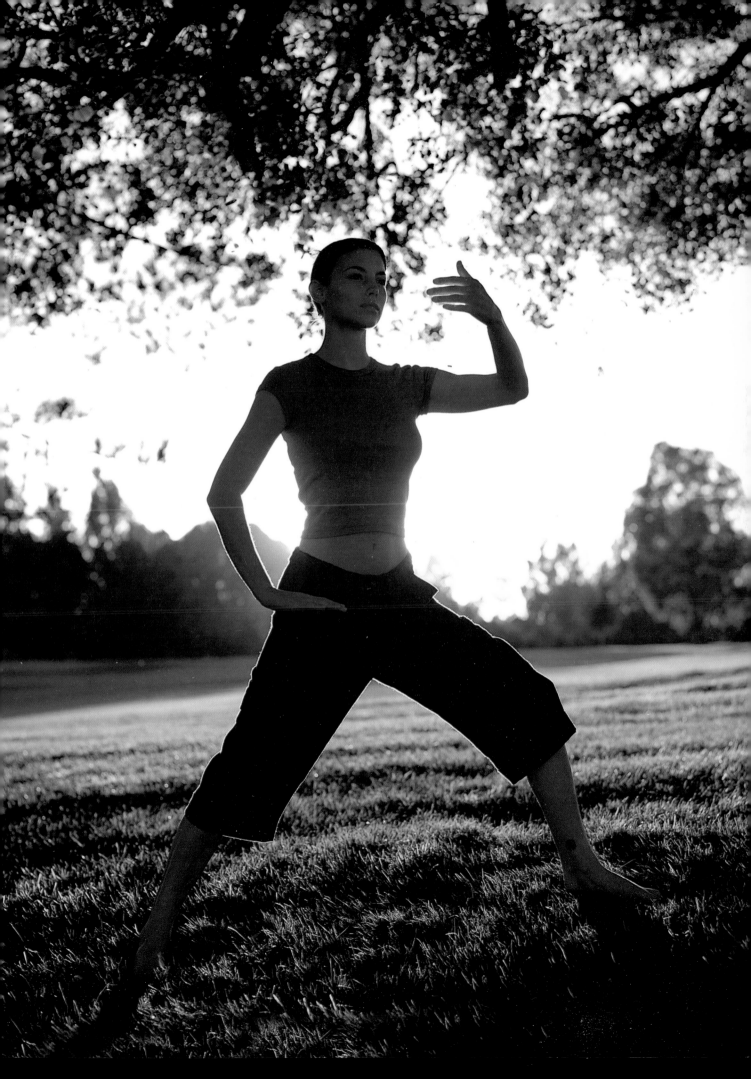

T'ai chi

It may originate in China, but t'ai chi has become a global form of movement therapy that is now almost as commonplace in Boston as it is in Beijing. Created in the thirteenth century by a Chinese Taoist monk, it is often described as an internal kung fu and aims to harness natural energy, both internally and externally. According to Taoist philosophy, chi (or life energy) has to flow freely through the body's energy channels or meridians, to prevent disease and to establish well being through balance. When the energy is blocked, illness can set in, so it's crucial that these pathways remain open.

These days, t'ai chi forms a staple part of the relaxation and well being programmes at many international spas. Not surprisingly, it has become as popular as yoga because of the potential health benefits if practised regularly. Don't expect to be huffing and puffing if you take up t'ai chi. It's a peaceful, elegant form of movement that is incredibly meditative to do.

Made up of a series of graceful arm movements and leg postures, each movement symbolizes the process of harnessing the energy around us and drawing it into the body. The movements are performed in sequence that at advanced levels comprises 108 over a thirty-minute session. The sequence given here can but only touch on the full effect.

At spas such as the Ojai Valley Inn and Spa and the Golden Door, both in California, USA, t'ai chi is one of the most popular relaxation techniques on the menu. There are many forms of t'ai chi from yang taijiquan to zenon wudang t'ai chi chuan, featured here.

The t'ai chi chuan sequence

This sequence has been adapted by Michael Jacques of T'ai Chi UK and represents the zenon wudang ta'i chi chuan system.

GUIDELINES
• Although t'ai chi chuan is very gentle and safe, it is wise to have a medical check-up before you start, especially if you do suffer from a specific medical condition.
• Dress in loose, comfortable clothing. You don't need to wear shoes if training indoors. But if you are training outside, wear well-fitting shoes with cushioned, flexible soles and arch supports. Your toes should be able to move freely.
• T'ai chi chuan can be practised at home, in a large room, in a park or your garden. Ideally, you should join a class or find an instructor to learn the form correctly.
• You will get more benefits from t'ai chi chuan if you practise daily. Increase the amount of time you spend practising as you become accustomed to the system.
• The more you practise, the better you will get and the more benefits you will gain. You will become mentally alert but relaxed, your mood will improve and your confidence and self-esteem will be boosted.
• Regular practice has also been shown to improve the following ailments: diabetes mellitus (late onset), peripheral vascular disease, mild high blood pressure, asthma and arthritis.

THE T'AI CHI MOVES

T'ai chi at rest

1 With your arms by your sides, palms down, and feet shoulder-width apart, bend your wrists, relax and breathe normally (a).

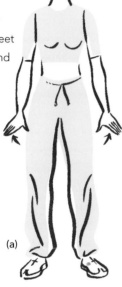

(a)

T'ai chi ready style stance

2 Relax, with your hands down by your sides (b).

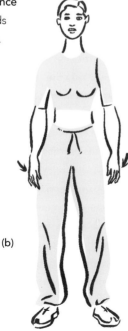

(b)

T'ai chi beginning style

3 Inhale and raise your arms in front of you to shoulder height.
4 Bend your arms and bring your hands to your shoulders.
5 Lower your arms.
6 Bend your knees and sink down.
7 Transfer all the weight to your right leg and then step forwards on to your left heel.
8 Bring your left arm in front of you so that the palm faces the chest (c).
9 Bring your right arm in front of you so that the right palm faces the left.
10 Turn your left foot in so that the sole is flat parallel to the ground.
11 Transfer your weight to your front leg by bending your left knee and straightening your right leg (d).

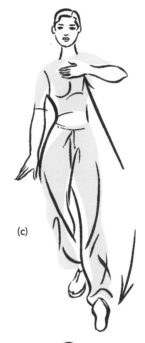

(c)

Seven stars style

12 Following on from the last position, reach out to the right with your right arm.
13 Keep your position, raise your right heel and turn your body to the right.
14 Bring your left fingers in contact with your right wrist and step forwards on to your right heel.

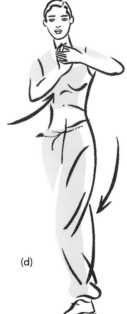

(d)

Yoga

Practised in India for over three thousand years, yoga is increasingly popular and relevant to modern day living. Yoga provides an effective antidote to the stresses that most of us suffer, combining spiritual, physical and mental disciplines that aim to maintain the balance of mind, body and spirit. To understand the scope of yoga and the effects produced, a six-day programme has been designed at The Spa at Rajvilas, Jaipur, India. It includes basic poses, breathing exercises and relaxation techniques. Also included is a detoxifying programme aimed at cleansing the systems of the body. At the end of the programme, the aim is to:

• Have a rejuvenated and re-energised body.
• Get initiated into a logical philosophy of a healthier lifestyle.
• Develop self-discipline.
• Become aware of the self and the physical body.
• Become more aware of and responsive to the surroundings.
• Learn to relax.

(The programme is not intended for those who suffer from medical conditions. In such cases, please seek advice of an experienced teacher/doctor.)

The programme's benefits are optimised if it is coupled with detoxifying changes in the diet. Abstain from alcohol, tobacco, tea, coffee, non-vegetarian food, onion, garlic and aerated drinks. They produce toxins, which may inhibit the efficient functions of the body's systems. As a yogic lifestyle is closely associated to ayurveda, the intake of these foods, which act as stimulants producing tamasic (gross) effects in the body, must be abstained from.

Mild withdrawal symptoms such as headache, nausea and diarrhoea may be experienced. These symptoms also denote that detoxification is taking place within your bodily system. All the same, if any of the symptoms persist for more than two days, please consult an experienced teacher/doctor. The postures overleaf are chosen because they help to achieve equilibrium for both the physical body and the bio-energies at a subtler level. They may help in quitting or reducing quite considerably the intake of caffeine, nicotine and alcohol and an awareness of breathing reduces stress levels.

GUIDELINES

• It is advisable while following the programme to have light meals with an increased intake of water, milk, juices, fresh vegetables and fruits. There should be a period of at least four to five hours between a meal and the yoga session.
• Practise yoga in a clean, quiet, well-ventilated environment. Though the preference of time differs with each of us, practise whenever you are not in a hurry.
• Clothing should be light and comfortable and should not hinder the movements of your body.
• You will need two blankets and one non-slip mattress to perform these postures.
• A light snack of milk with fruits is suggested after an hour of each session.

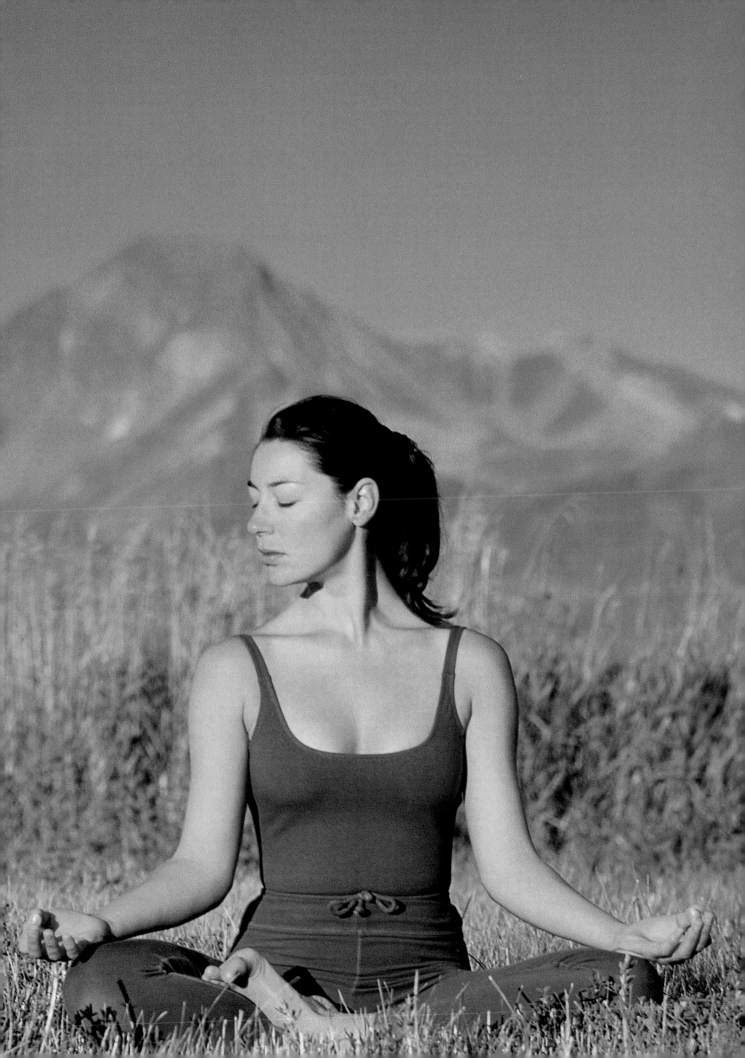

The yogic rejuvenation programme

from The Spa at Rajvilas, Jaipur, India

DAY 1

Breathing check (general)

Lie down on your back as comfortably as possible, leaving your whole body relaxed. Close your eyes and become aware of your breathing. After 2 to 3 minutes, put your right hand on your stomach. Now observe the movement of the hand. With each inhalation your hand should rise and with each exhalation, it should fall.

Sukhasana (easy pose)

This pose is performed by sitting cross-legged and with your eyes open. Sit on a folded blanket, with your legs crossed over the mattress and at the shins. Your spine and the neck are slightly extended; the shoulders slightly pulled back. Your body weight is evenly supported; breathing is slow, smooth and effortless (a). Become aware of your physical body and your surroundings. Hold the pose for 2 to 3 minutes. Slowly straighten your legs and relax for a moment; re-cross, changing the position of the legs. Hold for 2 to 3 minutes. Repeat the whole set once.

(a)

Vajrasana (rock pose)

Perform this movement by kneeling down with your knees kept together and sitting, evenly balancing your body between the calves and the heels. Your spine and neck are kept straight and the shoulders are even. Keep the eyes open and become aware of your body and the surroundings. Breathe slowly and smoothly. Hold for 2 to 3 minutes. Repeat once after relaxing the legs for a minute.

Bhadrasna (rock pose variant)

Sit in the rock pose as performed before but this time slowly cross your hands behind your back at the lower back level and with your eyes open. Bend your neck forwards and fix your gaze between the knees at an imaginary point. Feel the expansion of your chest and shoulders with each inhalation. Hold for 2 to 3 minutes. Repeat once after resting the legs for 1 minute.

   Caution: in case of neck pain or cervical spondylitis, do not bend your neck. Keep it straight and gaze at an imaginary point at eye level.

Makarasana (crocodile pose)

Lie flat on your stomach on a mattress with your arms stretched above your head and with your chin on the mattress; give a slight stretch to the body, keeping the big toes together. Fix your gaze between your hands. Hold for 2 to 3 minutes.

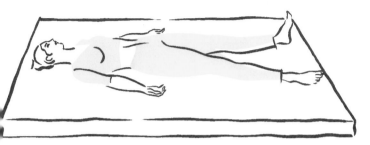

(b)

Shavasana (corpse pose)

Slowly turn over to lie down on your back, with your eyes closed. Let your whole body's weight be on the mattress. Slowly become aware of your body. Let your legs, trunk, shoulders, arms and neck become loose (b). Become aware of your breathing, inhale slowly and smoothly; exhale the same way. Observe the rise and the fall of your stomach. Relax in this position for 10 to 12 minutes. Then get up slowly.

DAY 2

Tadasana (palm tree pose)

This is a static pose in which you stand with your big toes and ankles together. Your spine and neck are extended slightly and shoulders slightly pulled back. Let your arms hang loose at your sides. The body is kept balanced on your feet while maintaining the whole posture evenly. Fix your gaze at an imaginary point straight ahead. Breathe slowly and smoothly. Maintain this pose for 30 to 60 seconds and repeat twice.

Caution: do not jump into the pose and do not over extend your knees.

Vriksasana (the tree pose)

Stand in tadasana. Slowly raise your left leg sideways, bend it at the knee and position the foot on the top of your inner left thigh. Slowly raise your arms and stretch them above the head joining the palms (c). Fix your gaze at an imaginary point straight ahead. Breathe slowly and smoothly. Maintain for 30 to 60 seconds. Repeat, alternating the legs. Repeat the set.

Caution: do not jump into the pose and do not overbalance on one foot; keep it firmly on the floor. Do not over extend your knees.

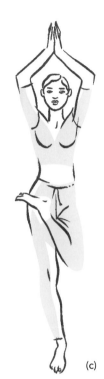

(c)

Ashwathasana (the peepul tree pose)

Stand in tadasana and raise your left arm straight above your head and the right one towards the side, palm downwards. Gradually stretch your right leg backwards without bending the knee and maintain the pose for 30 to 60 seconds. Repeat, alternating the position of your hands and legs. Repeat the set.

Caution: do not jump into the pose and do not overbalance on one foot; keep it firmly on the floor. Do not over extend your knees.

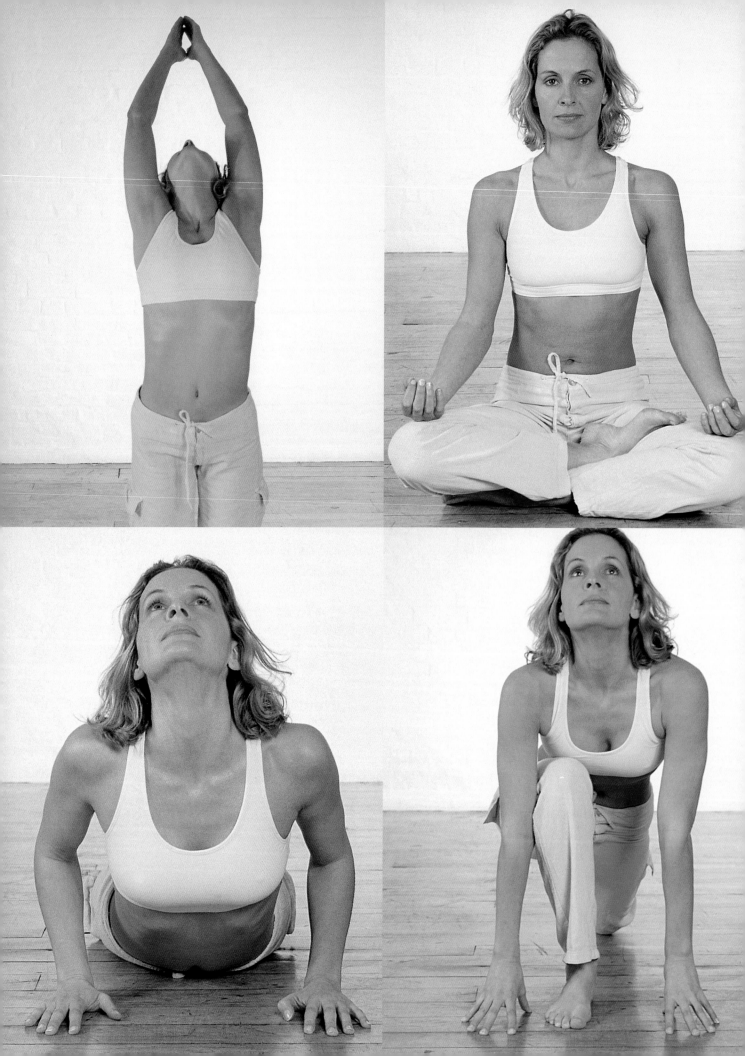

Veerasana (hero's pose)

Stand in tadasana and stretch your right leg backwards. Rest the right knee on the floor so that the left leg is bent at the knee. Raise your arms parallel to your shoulders in front of your body and clench the fists. Slowly straighten your right leg so that the weight is on the left leg. Extend the left arm and flex the right one so that your elbow touches your waist. Hold for 60 to 90 seconds. Repeat, alternating the position of the legs and the arms. Repeat the set.

Shavasana (corpse pose)

Slowly turn over to lie down on your back, with your eyes closed. Let your whole body's weight be on the mattress. Slowly become aware of your body. Let your legs, trunk, shoulders, arms and neck become loose. Become aware of your breathing, inhale slowly and smoothly; exhale the same way. Observe the rise and the fall of your stomach. Relax in this position for 10 to 12 minutes. Then get up slowly.

DAY 3

Repeat the poses done on Days 1 and 2 except for shavasana, a longer version of which is given below for finishing your yoga exercises for Day 3.

On Day 3 for all the seated poses, keep your eyes closed; breathe as in shavasana, slowly and smoothly and visualise your body being enveloped in a warm aura of energy. Repeat each pose three times, holding each for 2 to 3 minutes.

For all the standing poses, keep your eyes open; breathe as in shavasana; keep your gaze fixed and visualise your body as it appears in the pose. Feel the energies of the body getting balanced and flowing throughout the body.

Repeat all poses three times, holding each between 30 and 90 seconds.

Shavasana (corpse pose)

Lie down on your back, with your eyes closed. Let the whole body's weight be on the mattress. Slowly become aware of your body. Let your legs, trunk, shoulders, arms and neck become loose. Become aware of your breathing, inhale slowly and smoothly; exhale the same way. Observe the rise and the fall of your stomach. Inhale normally and exhale smoothly and slowly without straining yourself; let the exhalation be longer than the inhalation. Relax and keep the breathing rhythm for 5 to 6 minutes. Stay in the shavasana for 10 to 12 minutes.

THE LONG-TERM BENEFITS OF YOGA

• Regular practice of yoga has been shown to improve oxygen supply to the blood, thereby benefiting the circulation.

• Since yoga focuses on carefully balanced stretches and postures, there tends to be less risk of joint problems.

• Deeper breathing helps to reduce conditions such as asthma and can reduce the likelihood of panic attacks and hyperventilation.

• Conditions such as constipation are also alleviated as yogic breathing and postures help to stimulate the digestive system.

• Yoga helps to reduce blood pressure, stress-related headaches and back pain caused by tension and poor posture.

Aikido

According to Daintree spa's resident ki aikido specialist, Roby Kessler, regular practice of these Japanese exercises helps to bring harmony and vitality to our lives. Not only do they promote physical and mental health in the individual, but they also influence our daily interactions with others. 'Ki is the universal energy that can be directed through the mind, which then affects the body. (You may have heard the saying: Where the mind goes the body will follow),' says Kessler.

Ki development was founded in the early twentieth century by Morihei Ueshiba. Koichi Tonei, who was Ueshiba's chief instructor, went on to espouse the fundamental ki aikido principles:

1 Ki is extending.
2 Know your opponent's mind.
3 Respect your opponent's ki.
4 Put yourself in your opponent's place.
5 Lead with confidence.

A beginner's ki aikido course

from Daintree Eco-Lodge and Spa, Queensland, Australia

Supporting the Daintree Eco Lodge philosophy that mind/body connection influences good health, staff and guests are invited to participate in morning ki aikido sessions. Like t'ai chi and yoga, aikido is best learnt from a qualified instructor. However, Roby Kessler has devised a beginner's course that you can practise at home.

GUIDELINES

• The following stretching exercises serve to unify the mind and body when in motion.
• Perform the movements in a fluid and comfortable manner.
• Remember to keep your mind and body unified by following any one of the following principles: keep centred; relax completely; keep your weight underside (where the weight naturally falls) or extend ki – do what you do with 100 percent focus.
• Work in an open space, preferably at a comfortable room temperature.
• Wear loose, warm clothing.
• Put on some music of your choice, preferably soft with a slight beat.

TOITSU-TAISO (COORDINATION EXERCISES)

Trunk twist
Stand with your feet apart and slightly parallel (shoulder length distance between them) and twist the trunk from side to side by swinging the arms (a).
Left: count 1-2; Right: count 3-4; Left: count 5-6; Right: count 7-8. Perform twice.

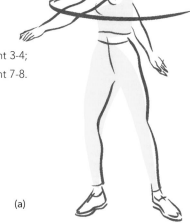

(a)

Bend the trunk to the side

Left: count 1-2; Right: count 3-4; Left: count 5-6; Right: count 7-8.
Perform twice.

Bend forwards and backwards (knees bent)

Forwards: count 1-2; Backwards: count 3-4; Forwards: count 5-6; Backwards: count 7-8. Perform twice (b and c).

(b)

(c)

Shoulder blade exercise

Bend your arms in front of you and then raise your elbows so that they are parallel with the floor, then gently push left shoulder back, then right shoulder back twice.
Left: count 1-2; Right: count 3-4; Left: count 5-6; Right: count 7-8.
Perform twice.

Neck stretches

Bend the neck from side to side, with each ear moving towards the corresponding shoulder blade. Repeat. Then move your head backwards and forwards. Repeat, Finally, carefully bend the neck from front to back in a controlled manner. Repeat.
Left: count 1-2; Right: count 3-4; Left: count 5-6; Right: count 7-8.

Arm swings 1

Standing upright with feet slightly apart, swing one arm (forward swing only) at a time.
Left: count 1-2-3-4; Right: count 5-6-7-8.
Perform twice.

Arm swings 2

Swing both arms (d).
Forwards: count 1-2-3-4; Backwards: count 5-6-7-8.
Perform twice.

Arm swings 3

Now swing both arms while gently bending the knees.
Forwards: count 1-2-3-4; Backwards: count 5-6-7-8.
Perform twice.

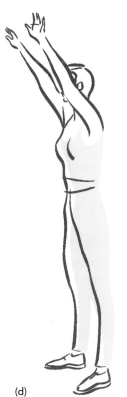

(d)

Meditation

Once upon a time, we Westerners viewed meditation with scepticism. It was practised either by Eastern gurus who spent their lives in isolation in search of Nirvana and enlightenment or adopted by neo-hippies as a legal way of 'getting high'. How times have changed. Now considered by many as commonplace as aromatherapy, some forms of meditation such as transcendental meditation are even recommended by GPs as an effective solution for stress-related conditions. At health spas east and west, you are just as likely to find meditation on the menu as you are aerobic and stretch classes. The reason? Regular practice of a meditation technique has been proven to lower blood pressure, lessen our risk of developing certain diseases, including cancer, and to generally boost our immune system. Not only that, it is a sure-fire way of allowing us to tune in to our natural state of tranquillity.

The Expanding Light yoga and meditation retreat was founded over 27 years ago in the Sierra Nevada foothills of northern California.

THE BENEFITS OF MEDITATION

• Meditation significantly controls high blood pressures at levels comparable to widely used prescription drugs, without the side effects.
• Chronic pain can be reduced by more than 50 percent.
• 75 percent of long-term insomniacs who have been trained in meditation can fall asleep within 20 minutes of going to bed.
• Meditation decreases oxygen consumption, heart rate, respiratory rate and blood pressure, and increases the intensity of alpha, theta and delta brain waves – the opposite of the physiological changes that occur during the stress response.
• Meditators have been shown to be less anxious and neurotic, more spontaneous, independent, self-confident, empathetic and less fearful of death.

Famed for their yoga and meditation workshops, devotees travel from far and wide to learn the art of tranquillity in this truly peaceful retreat. Based on the universal teachings of the great Indian master, Paramhansa Yogananda, author of the spiritual classic, *Autobiography of a Yogi*, the workshops recognise that everyone's path is unique, that true spiritual growth should benefit every aspect of your life, and that it comes from inner experience, not blind belief. The Expanding Light exists to support guests in their search.

So exactly what does meditation do for us? 'Meditation offers a wide variety of real benefits that have a deep-reaching impact on our lives,' explains Marilyn Carr, The Expanding Light's director. 'The meditator experiences greater peace, calmness and joy as the mind quiets and the heart expands. All areas of life – work, relationships and health – begin miraculously to change as the true Self comes home to itself.'

With regular practice, problems will be solved much more easily and your work will be done more quickly because your energies become more focused. You will also find that you can concentrate more deeply and act calmly in the face of difficult situations rather than reacting out of frustration or anger. 'Everything in life will, in time, look and feel different because it will be infused with that peace and joy which is our true nature,' adds Carr.

'It is not, as so many people assume it to be, a process of "thinking things over". Rather, it is making the mind completely receptive to reality. It is stilling the thought-processes – those restless ripples that bob on the surface of the mind – so that truth, like the moon, may be clearly reflected there. It is listening to God, to Universal Reality, for a change, instead of doing all the talking and "computing" oneself,' explains Carr.

HOW TO PRACTISE MEDITATION

At The Expanding Light at Ananda, meditation goes hand in hand with hatha yoga. For the best results, begin with perhaps half an hour of yoga postures or asanas and 15 minutes of meditation and increase the practices gradually as your mind and body are ready to do so. Instructions and guidelines are given here.

The ideal way to learn yoga and meditation would be on retreat from an experienced practitioner. This has many advantages, one being that you leave your daily concerns and tasks behind and can turn all of your attention to the incorporation of new practices into your life while being at a peaceful site that carries a vibration to support this new learning. It is important to carefully select such a place, one that feels right for you. The next best scenario would be to attend a local meditation and yoga workshop or course as these practices are most easily demonstrated visually by someone you can relate to personally. Then, as with the retreat option, you can incorporate the practices into your home routine.

If none of the above is possible in the near future, there's no need to wait. The instructions given overleaf can get you started on a powerful and transformative home practice. But read the following advice first.

GETTING COMFORTABLE FOR A SITTING MEDITATION

Before starting your meditation there are a few things that you can do to help the smooth flowing of your session.

Perform some yoga postures and energising exercises: yoga postures are a wonderful way to get the energy flowing. Or use other gentle exercises of your choice which calm, rather than excite, the nervous system.

Say a prayer: always ask for guidance. Say a prayer mentally or out loud in whatever form that feels comfortable to you. Don't forget this important step.

Do some chanting: if you don't play a musical instrument, have a chanting tape to sing along with, either out loud or mentally. Chanting opens the heart, an important ingredient for deep meditation.

Sit comfortably: one of the most important aspects of a sitting meditation is to be able to sit comfortably, without suffering an aching back, legs that hurt or going to sleep. If you are in pain or great discomfort, the only thing you will be meditating on is that! The options for sitting are in a chair, on a meditation bench or on a pillow on the floor. Most Westerners are not trained from birth to sit comfortably on a hard floor. So a chair is probably best for most of us, beginners or otherwise, and many very great meditators with many years experience use a chair or stool for their meditations. It is not a sign of lack of meditative ability if you are unable to sit in the lotus posture or any other floor sitting position.

Get a fairly straight-backed chair and sit forward in the chair so that both feet are flat on the floor. If your feet do not touch the floor, get a shorter chair or place a pillow or two under your feet to raise them so that your thighs are parallel to the floor. Do not lean against the back of the chair. The idea is to sit with an upright, unsupported spine. However, if you are not used to sitting this way, or if you have weak neck/back muscles or injuries, there are ways to overcome

PRACTICAL HINTS FOR MEDITATION

Regularity: set aside the same time or times each day for your meditation. Recommended times are dawn (just after awakening), twilight, high noon and midnight. Another is in the evening, just before bedtime. It is best always to meditate on an empty stomach (2-3 hours after meals).

Location: set aside a room, or small part of a room, just for meditation. Try to find as quiet a spot as possible or, if this is difficult, try using comfortable foam earplugs or headphones to block out noise. Be sure the room is not stuffy and that it is a bit on the cool side; a blanket or shawl to wrap up in is nice. Have a place to sit, and a small, simple altar or focal point, like pictures, flowers and candles. You will find that the vibrations of meditation build here. If possible, face east. Yogis say that there are certain natural currents that flow east to west, which help you meditate better.

Say a little prayer: upon beginning your meditation, say a prayer either out loud, or inwardly, to God and the Masters, to guide and help you. It is also helpful to do some chanting, if you can (using a cassette tape of chants is very nice – sing along with it!).

Meditate with joy, with devotion: don't wait for God's joy to make you joyful, be joyful first yourself! Meditation simply helps you remember, on deepening levels of awareness, who and what you really are. You are a child of God; you are one with the infinite Light.

Use a blanket or two: many yogis recommend sitting on a wool rug, blanket, or piece of silk. Also the place you meditate should be a little on the cool side with a source of fresh air if possible. Thus another blanket or warm meditation shawl should be handy to wrap up in. The body does cool down when you sit still for a while, so a wrap is often important to maintain an even body temperature. Get comfortable, but stay awake and ready!

this challenge. Get a firm pillow of some sort (the crescent shaped ones are very good for this) and put it between your back and the back of the chair. The feeling you want is that of support, but not leaning into it. Move the pillow around until you achieve this feeling. If you want to place a pillow in the seat of the chair, to cushion a too hard surface, that is fine.

Meditate for short periods of time in the beginning and work up to longer amounts of time. In this way, your back muscles will strengthen gradually. Yoga stretches and other such exercises also strengthen your back muscles with time and regular practice. Do not set unrealistic goals for yourself. It is better to meditate for 5 to 15 minutes and be consistent about it, and then increase your time as you can. One longer meditation each week is very helpful.

Meditation benches are a wonderful invention for making the legs feel comfortable and un-pressured and keeping the spine upright. Finding the right size and height is important. Padding on the seat often helps. Adding small pillows under the knees or ankles might facilitate your comfort also. If you have never tried a bench, please be sure to experiment with one. Some people are more comfortable sitting cross-legged on a pillow. You can buy crescent-shaped or round-plump pillows, which are designed to help with this position.

So experiment. Have a chair, lots of pillows, a bench and whatever else you want to try. When one position becomes tiresome, calmly switch to another. Eventually you'll find the best one for your body-type. Remember, everybody's body is different. You should feel relatively relaxed once you have finished meditating but sitting on the wrong chair or without sufficient pillows will make this state more difficult to achieve.

The Hong-Sau technique of meditation

from The Expanding Light, California, USA

The breath and mind react intimately upon one another. The breath instantly responds to different mental and emotional states. As the breath flows, so flows the mind. By concentrating on the breath, the mind becomes calmer. This is the Hong-Sau technique of concentration and meditation as taught by Paramhansa Yogananda and also by his disciple, Swami Kriyananda, the founder and spiritual director of The Expanding Light, and it is this technique that is described here.

1 Energisation, prayer, and chanting are suggested before meditation, but Hong-Sau actually may be done at any time and in any place. If you have time, exercise a little before meditation. Yoga postures are excellent and, of course, Yogananda's energisation exercises are highly recommended. Remember that the exercises you do before meditation should calm, not excite, the nervous system.

2 Inhale and tense the whole body. Exhale and relax. Repeat three times. Then, inhale slowly to a count of 6 to 10; hold the breath to that same count; exhale to that count and immediately inhale again to the same count. Repeat 6 to 10 times. Please remember that these are preliminary breathing exercises, not the technique itself.

3 Now, without counting or tension, take a long, slow, deep breath. When the breath begins to flow again, begin to observe its movement, without any attempt to control it. Notice the place at which you can observe the breath in your body whether in the lungs, in the nostrils or sinuses. Be an impartial observer, not caring whether it flows in or out or remains stationary. Simply remain attentive to whatever the breath does by itself, naturally. Moving the forefinger of the right hand in for inhalation and out for exhalation may be helpful for helping you tune into the breath.

4 Follow the inhalation with the mantra Hong (pronounced to rhyme with song) and the exhalation with the mantra Sau (pronounced like saw). Repeat the mantra mentally only. Be careful not to move the lips or tongue. Hong-Sau is a Sanskrit mantra meaning 'I am He' or 'I am Spirit'.

5 As your practice deepens, begin to enjoy the pauses between the inhalations and the exhalations, when the breath is not flowing. Do not actively hold the breath in or out. As many times as your mind wanders away from Hong-Sau, bring it gently back to the technique.

6 After your period of practice of this technique (5 to 10 minutes is fine for beginners, gradually increasing the time as you go) inhale and exhale three times, and then leave the breath out for as long as is comfortable for you. Then begin breathing normally once again.

7 Throughout the practice, keep your eyes closed and looking upward towards the point between the eyebrows; don't strain your eyes – let them relax!

8 After completing your practice of Hong-Sau, be sure to sit in silence and stillness for at least as long as you practised the technique. Practise devotion, inward chanting, visualisation or prayer. Hold your body still and be very silent and relaxed, yet aware.

May the powerful meditation/concentration technique of Hong-Sau bring you ever closer to your own highest potential.

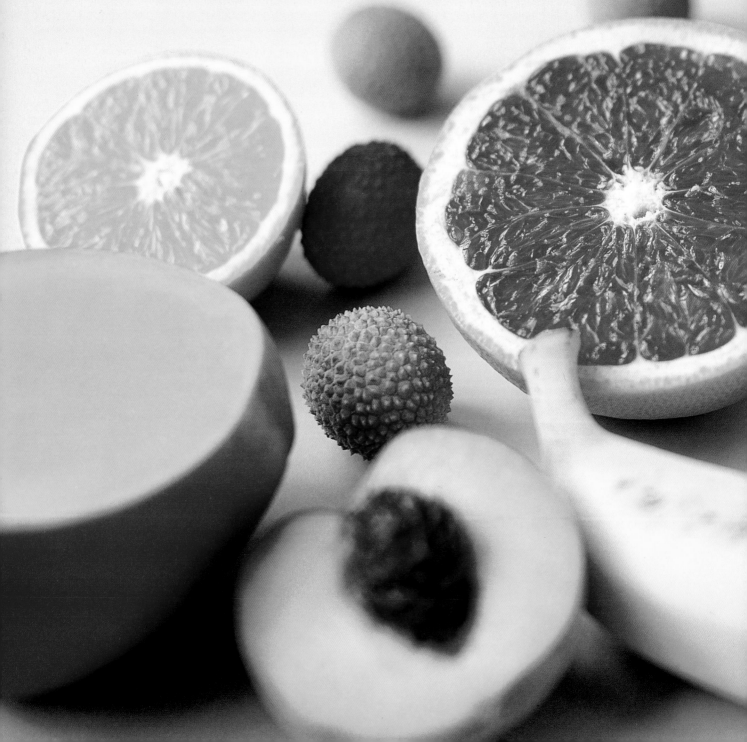

eat THE SPA WAY TO health

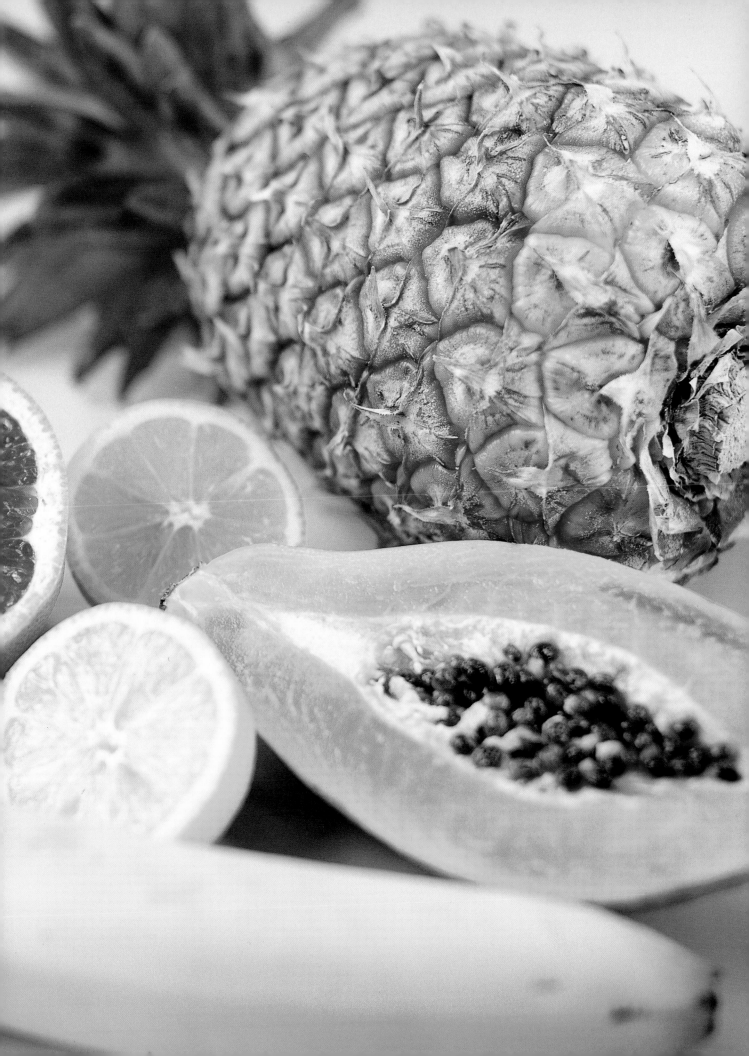

The spa food philosophy

When it comes to eating well, nobody's perfect. Even nutritionists and health gurus more than occasionally forget to practise what they preach, swigging the odd glass of champagne and skipping meals from time to time. No one wants to be dictated to when it comes to what we eat but we all know that apart from the incredibly virtuous, our diets could be better. As well as the obvious fact that sometimes 'bad' things are too good to resist, the main reason that most of us go off the rails, whether once in a while or perpetually, is down to lifestyle. It's all too easy when we are feeling fractious and fatigued to forget about health food and load up on junk food.

Be it late-night takeaways or fast food grabbed on the run, we are constantly depriving ourselves of freshly prepared meals that are nutrient-rich, not to mention delicious. While we can't always book in to a spa to re-educate our palette and de-toxify our body, we can benefit from culinary spa know-how at home. I've gathered some of the best recipes from premier spas around the world so that you can create your own home-spa food programme. You can use it as a once in a while de-tox and to boost vital nutrients or you might be completely converted and never return to convenience and fast foods again.

The philosophy behind spa food is simple, not to mention universal. It is designed to feed your body on all levels, with colours and textures that are visually appealing and tastes and aromas that satisfy, stimulate and cleanse. Contrary to popular belief, the food served up at modern spas and health resorts does not consist of a few meagre bean sprouts or a bowl of mushy gruel,

as some of my non-spa-going friends seem to think. It can be as delicious and sophisticated as anything you might find on any haute cuisine menu anywhere in the world. First-class chefs are employed to create tantalising food that also has a healthy spin. It's obvious that low fat, salt and sugar is the order of the day – but that doesn't mean the food tastes bland. Far from it, as I hope you will find out from first-hand experience.

SIMPLE GUIDELINES FOR BALANCE

The secret to eating healthily – no surprises here – is balance. Whether you're cooking at home, dining out or choosing a takeaway on the run, here are a few tips from the experts at Canyon Ranch, Arizona, USA.

Fruits and vegetables: every meal should include fruits or vegetables, and preferably both. If you make these foods the central component of a meal, you won't overlook them. Research has shown that a diet rich in fruits and vegetables is rich in disease-fighting nutrients such as antioxidants and phytochemicals. Try to include five to nine servings from this food group every day by including them in soups, salads, sandwich filings, stir-fries and juices.

Carbohydrate-rich foods: this category includes beans, soybeans, peas, corn, potatoes, brown and wild rice and grains including barley and millet, and breads and pasta made from any of these grains. Being rich in carbohydrates and fibre, they also include some protein. Make sure you get plenty of variety and don't just end up sticking to white breads and pasta. Keep to moderately sized portions.

Protein-rich foods: fish, poultry, soy foods, beans, eggs, low-fat dairy foods, nuts, seeds and lean meat. These foods are the most concentrated sources of protein and including them in a meal will help to satisfy hunger and sustain energy levels.

Fat: at Canyon Ranch and many other spas, it is suggested that about 20 percent of our total calorie intake comes from fat. You may need to tailor this to your own preferences and health conditions. It means that you should be eating about 25-40 g of fat a day from the healthiest sources, which include extra virgin olive oil, canola oil, olives, nuts, seeds, avocados and fatty fish like salmon and tuna. It is a wise idea to avoid as much hydrogenated fat as possible, usually found in margarine, biscuits and ready prepared popcorn. Don't cut out fat completely, though, unless your doctor has advised you to.

Fibre: low-fat diets can be low in fibre because they are centred around white flour products like bagels and pasta. You should get 25-40 g of dietary fibre each day in the form of bran cereal, whole grains, beans, fruits and vegetables. Not only does fibre help to maintain blood sugar levels, it lowers cholesterol levels and, furthermore, helps to keep the digestive system in peak condition. New research has also suggested that fibre influences hormone levels and affects the immune system.

Salt and sugar: try to keep salt intake to a minimum, particularly if you suffer from high blood pressure. If you do use salt, choose natural sea salt. As for sugar, most spas try to limit the use of refined sugar, opting instead for molasses, honey, fruit juice concentrate and fructose.

Water: most nutritionists advocate drinking at least eight glasses a day. The general consensus is that water is essential to dilute the waste materials excreted by the body. This ensures that kidneys are not over-worked and it prevents dehydration. Coffee and tea are not water substitutes. In fact, caffeinated beverages are diuretics and only serve to further dehydrate your body. If you are addicted to hot drinks, swap to herbal tisanes, or try a little lemon juice and honey in hot water as a tea or coffee replacement.

SPA COOKING TIPS
• Use plenty of herbs and spices. As they contain practically no calories, they can be used liberally to flavour foods. Sprinkle them on salads and in soups to replace salt and compensate for fat.
• Use non-stick pots and pans. Cut down on your use of oil by cooking everything from fish, poultry and pancakes in non-stick cookware.
• Cook or roast at a low temperature for a longer period of time. Using slow-cookers or roasting in an oven at a very low temperature helps flavours to marry and creates a rich-tasting dish with little or no fat.

Breakfast

Most nutritionists consider that breakfast is the most important meal of the day, yet many of us tend to skip it because we're just in too much of a hurry. Make an effort to include a satisfying nutritious breakfast each day, even if it's only for one week once a month. You don't need to spend hours preparing it – a simple feast of fresh fruit and yoghurt, wholegrain bread and a herbal tea will set you up for the day ahead.

Grilled banana with cashew nuts and honey served with fresh fruit

from the Nusa Dua Spa, Bali, Indonesia
Makes 4 servings

4 bananas
60 ml honey
25 g chopped cashew nuts
125 ml plain yoghurt
60 ml orange juice
2 tsp dextrose
4 sticks lemon grass or wooden kebab sticks
75 g chopped papaya
50 g chopped watermelon
25 g grapefruit segments

1 Slice the bananas in half and grill until they are a little soft.
2 Brush with honey and sprinkle with the chopped cashew nuts.
3 Grill again until golden brown.
4 Combine the yoghurt, orange juice and dextrose. Then arrange the fresh fruit on the plates and pour the yoghurt-orange mix around the edge.
5 Skewer the bananas on a lemon grass or wooden stick, pile on top of the fruit and serve.

Granola

from Rancho La Puerta, Baja California, Mexico
Makes 6 servings

350 g old-fashioned rolled oats
50 g chopped almonds
75 g sunflower seeds
25 g wholewheat flour
25 g oat bran
1 tbsp ground cinnamon
¾ tsp ground ginger
1 tsp cardamom
175 ml honey
125 ml unsweetened, unfiltered apple juice
2 tbsp vanilla extract
2 tsp canola oil
2 tsp grated orange zest
2 tbsp fresh orange juice (optional)

1 Preheat the oven to 130°C/250°F/Gas Mark ½. Lightly coat a baking sheet with vegetable oil spray.
2 In a large mixing bowl, combine the rolled oats, almonds, seeds, flour, oat bran, cinnamon, ginger and cardamom.
3 In another bowl, whisk together the honey, apple juice, vanilla and oil until the honey is thoroughly incorporated. Add the orange zest and the orange juice, if desired.
4 Pour the wet ingredients over the dry ingredients and mix well. Spread the granola evenly over the baking sheet and bake for 1½ hours, checking every 15 minutes. When the granola starts to brown, stir gently with a spatula. Take care that the outside edges do not burn. When golden and dry, scrape on to a plate or a cool baking sheet and set aside to cool. Store in an airtight container until ready to use.

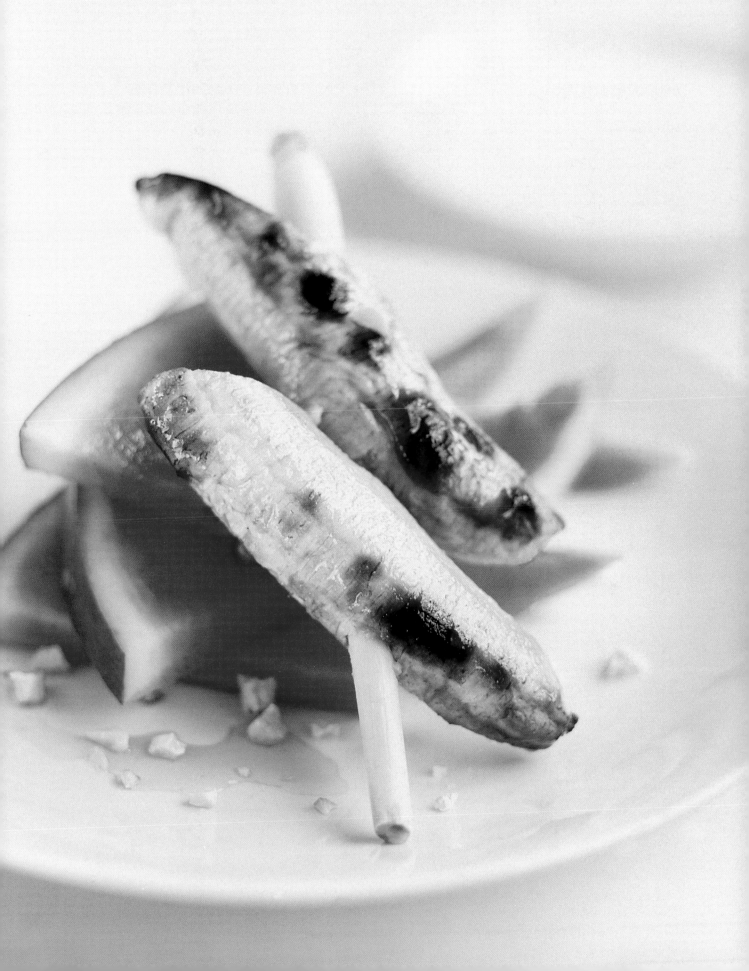

Alpine muesli

from Canyon Ranch, Arizona, USA
Makes 8 servings

50 g uncooked quick porridge oats
250 ml skimmed milk
125 ml plain non or low fat yoghurt
250 ml orange juice
35 g ground hazelnuts
60 ml fructose or honey
450 g apples, grated
450 g freshly chopped mixed fruits such as peach, apricot and melon.

1 In a large bowl, combine the oats, skimmed milk and yoghurt. Let it stand for 5 minutes to soften the oats.
2 Add the orange juice, ground nuts and fructose or honey. Stir thoroughly.
3 Grate the apple and stir into the mixture to prevent it browning. Stir in the chopped fruit. Serve chilled.

Oatmeal muesli bars

from Forest Mere Health Farm, Hampshire, UK
Makes 30 muesli bars

425 g plain flour
575 g oats
2½ tsp baking powder
300 g caster sugar
425 g margarine
5 tbsp honey
250 ml natural yoghurt

1 Put the flour, oats and baking powder into a mixing bowl.
2 Heat together very gently the sugar, margarine and honey.
3 When all the ingredients are melted together pour on to the oats and flour, adding the yoghurt too, and mix well until combined.
4 Add the flavourings (see below) and pour into a tray lined with greaseproof paper and spread evenly.
5 Bake at 150°C/300°F/Gas Mark 2 for 15 to 20 minutes.

IDEAS FOR FLAVOURINGS

Apple and date: put 150 g of dried apple and 50 g of dried stoned dates into a food mixer and pulse until roughly chopped. Add to the muesli mix before spreading on the baking tray.
Apricot and sunflower seed: put 200 g of dried apricots in a food mixer and pulse until roughly chopped, then add 100 g of sunflower seeds and add to the muesli mix as before.
Currant and pumpkin seed: add 200 g of currants and 100 g of pumpkin seeds to the muesli mix.
Prune and almond: add 200 g of pitted prunes and 150 g of flaked almonds to the mix.

Oatmeal

from the Golden Door, California, USA

Makes 4 servings

'Victoria Reynoso, who is in charge of breakfast at The Golden Door, revealed her secret for delicious oatmeal. Patience and a very low flame are their own reward. For the best flavour and texture, serve the oatmeal as soon as it thickens.' Michel Stroot, executive chef.

100 g old-fashioned rolled oats
¼ tsp salt (optional)
¼ tsp ground cinnamon
1 red or green apple, peeled, cored and grated
8 tsp honey
25 g raisins or currants

1 In a medium sized saucepan, bring 450 ml of water to the boil over a high heat. Add the oats, the salt, if desired, and the cinnamon. Stir once, reduce the heat to low and simmer, uncovered, for 5 minutes without stirring.
2 Add the grated apple and simmer for a further 5 to 7 minutes, stirring only once or twice, until the oatmeal is quite thick. Remove from the heat, cover and let stand for 10 minutes until very thick.
3 Spoon into warmed bowls, drizzle with the honey and top each serving with a sprinkling of the raisins.

Oatbran pancakes with warm peach sauce

From the Wyndham Resort and Spa, Florida, USA

Makes 2 servings

50 g unprocessed oat bran
25 g wholewheat flour
2 tsp baking powder
2 tsp sugar
1 tbsp water
25 g mashed banana
2 egg whites
125 ml plain non-fat yoghurt
orange slices and strawberry fans to garnish

Warm peach sauce
175 ml unsweetened peach conserves
175 ml unsweetened apple juice
1 tsp cornflour

1 In a medium bowl, combine the bran, flour, baking powder and sugar. In a small bowl, stir the water, mashed banana, egg whites and yoghurt until well combined. Pour into the oat bran mixture and stir.
2 Spray a non-stick frying pan or griddle with vegetable oil and place over a medium heat. Pour in 125 ml of the batter for each pancake, allowing room for spreading. Cook until the sides are brown and bubbles form around the edges. Turn and cook until the bottoms are light brown.
3 For the sauce, heat the peach conserves in a small saucepan over low heat. In a cup, stir the apple juice and cornflour until smooth. Add to the conserves. Bring to the boil, stirring frequently.
4 To serve, place half of the pancakes on each of two plates. Top with the Warm Peach Sauce and garnish with oranges and strawberry fans.

Potato and chive cakes with poached eggs and smoked salmon

from Champneys, Hertfordshire, UK

Makes 4 servings

250 g cooked mashed potato
50 g wholemeal flour
3 tbsp chopped chives
1 tsp crushed coriander seeds
salt and freshly ground black pepper
1 tbsp groundnut or grapeseed oil
1 tbsp white wine vinegar
4 eggs
4 slices of smoked salmon
1 lemon, halved
flat leaf parsley to garnish

1 To make the potato cakes, mix the mashed potato with the flour, chives and crushed coriander seeds.
2 Season to taste with salt and pepper and mix to form a firm dough.
3 Roll out to a lightly floured surface to a thickness of 5 mm. Then, using a 7 cm cutter, cut out eight cakes.
4 Heat the oil in a non-stick frying pan and cook the potato cakes until lightly browned – about 3 minutes on each side.
5 Half fill a wide, shallow pan with water. Add the vinegar and bring to the boil. Reduce the heat to a gentle simmer and poach the eggs for 3 minutes or until softly poached. Lift out with a slotted spoon and drain on kitchen towel.
6 Serve two potato cakes per person with the poached eggs on top and a twist of smoked salmon on the side.
7 Grind black pepper and squeeze a little lemon over the salmon and garnish with parsley.

Blueberry muffins with an apple and cinnamon spread

from Ragdale Hall, Leicestershire, UK

Makes 6 muffins

100 g wholemeal flour
1 tsp baking powder
1 tbsp low-calorie sweetener
1 large egg, beaten
100 ml skimmed milk
50 g fresh blueberries
6 muffin tins

For the apple and cinnamon spread
2 large cooking apples
25 g unsalted low-fat spread
1 tsp clear honey
¼ tsp cinnamon

1 To prepare the muffins, sift the flour, baking powder and sweetener into a bowl.
2 Make a well in the centre and add the beaten egg and milk. Mix well, then carefully stir the blueberries into the muffin mixture, taking care not to break them up.
3 Divide the mixture into the muffin tins. Place in a preheated oven at 200°C/400°F/Gas Mark 6 and bake for 25 to 30 minutes.
4 While the muffins are baking, peel and core the apples and cook in a saucepan with a little water until soft. Drain off any excess water.
5 Melt the low-fat spread until runny and stir in the honey. Add the apples and cinnamon and blend the mixture for 20 seconds with a hand-held mixer until smooth.
6 Place the mixture into the refrigerator to chill and set.
7 Serve the muffins warmed, accompanied by the spread.

Lunch

Most spas share a common philosophy when it comes to food and that is that little and often is the best way of eating. The lunch and dinner recipes are, therefore, interchangeable. You may want to mix and match the soups and salads, have a lighter meal in the evening and a more satisfying lunch or vice versa – whatever suits your lifestyle, appetite and time constraints. Just bear in mind that variety is key and use the guidelines at the beginning of the chapter to ensure that you're getting sufficient quantities of the essential nutrients that your body requires.

Gazpacho soup

from Canyon Ranch, Arizona, USA
Makes 8 servings

1 large or 2 small tomatoes
75 g peeled diced cucumbers
100 g mixed diced red and green bell peppers
75 g diced onions
4 x 175 ml cans low-sodium V8 juice
½ tsp garlic powder
¼ tsp Worcestershire sauce
¼ tsp freshly ground black pepper
2 tbsp freshly squeezed lemon juice
chopped chives, to garnish
2 lemons, cut into 4 wedges

1 Bring a large pot of water to the boil. Cut a shallow cross in the top of the tomatoes with a sharp knife. Drop the tomatoes into boiling water for 2 minutes, then transfer to a bowl of iced water. Peel and dice. You should have 250 ml of tomatoes.
2 In a large bowl, combine all the ingredients except the garnish. Mix thoroughly and chill overnight.
3 Serve in chilled bowls and garnish with the chopped chives and the lemon wedges.

Watercress, endive and herb salad with garlic croutons and Parmesan in a cider dressing

from Henlow Grange Health Farm, Bedfordshire, UK
Makes 4 servings

For the dressing
1 egg
1 egg yolk
1 tbsp Dijon mustard
1 tbsp cider vinegar
500 ml vegetable oil
8 tbsp dry cider
salt and freshly ground black pepper
1 small baguette
garlic oil

2 bunches watercress
200 g curly endive salad
2 tbsp chopped mixed herbs (parsley, chervil, chives, basil and tarragon)
25 g Parmesan cheese, grated

1 Whisk the eggs with the mustard and vinegar and add the vegetable oil. As the dressing becomes too thick, thin with the cider. Season with salt and freshly ground black pepper.
2 To make chunky croutons, slice the baguette very thinly and lightly drizzle with garlic oil. Place into a hot oven and bake at 180°C/350°F/Gas Mark 4 until golden brown. Remove from the oven, season and leave to cool.
3 Take the watercress and endive and add the herbs, grated Parmesan cheese and garlic croutons. Coat with the dressing and serve.

Chicken and sugar snap pea stir-fry

from Echo Valley Ranch Resort, Jesmond, Canada
Makes 4 servings

2 tsp cornflour
1 tbsp low-salt soy sauce
160 ml chicken stock
2 tsp peanut oil
1 medium onion, chopped
1 medium red pepper, sliced
60 g sugar snap peas
500 g skinless chicken breast fillets, thinly sliced

1 Dissolve the cornflour in the soy sauce and add to the stock. Set aside. Heat half the oil in a wok, add the onion and pepper and stir-fry over a high heat until the onion is just soft.
2 Add the peas, stir-fry for a further minute, then remove the vegetables from the wok. Heat the remaining oil in the wok and stir-fry the chicken in batches until browned.
3 Return the vegetables to the wok and add the cornflour, stock and soy sauce until the mixture boils and thickens slightly.

Carrot and raisin salad

from Canyon Ranch, Arizona, USA
Makes 8 servings

50 g canned crushed pineapple with juice
6 tablespoons non-fat yogurt
6 tablespoons fat-free mayonnaise
1 kg carrots, grated
50 g raisins

1 Drain the pineapple, reserving the juice. Combine 3 tablespoons of the juice with the yoghurt and mayonnaise.
2 Add the pineapple and the carrots and raisins and mix well. Cover tightly and refrigerate until cold before serving.

Warm spinach dip with pita chips

from the Professional Golfers Association of America Resort and Spa, Florida, USA
Makes 8 servings

25 g diced onion
25 g diced artichoke hearts
2 tbsp chicken stock
100 g light cream cheese
125 ml non-fat sour cream
2 tbsp rice wine vinegar
ground black pepper
dash of hot pepper sauce
dash of Worcesershire sauce
50 g chopped fresh spinach
25 g diced spring onions
8 wholewheat pita breads, cut into quarters and toasted

1 In a large saucepan over medium heat, sauté the onion, artichoke hearts and chicken stock until the onions are translucent.
2 Add the cream cheese and the next five ingredients.
3 Bring to a simmer, stirring constantly.
4 Remove from the heat and stir in the spinach and spring onions.
5 Serve warm with toasted pita quarters.

Roasted red potato salad

from Rancho La Puerta, Baja California, Mexico

Makes 6 servings

2 tbsp balsamic vinegar

2 tbsp rice vinegar

2 garlic cloves, minced

½ tsp chopped fresh rosemary

pinch hot red pepper flakes (optional)

pinch freshly ground black pepper

½ tsp olive oil

4 large red potatoes, cut into 12 mm pieces

3 hard-boiled large egg whites, chopped

½ red onion, diced

1 celery stick, diced

1 medium tomato, diced

1 tsp minced fresh oregano

2 tbsp coarse-grain Dijon mustard

2 tbsp non-fat plain yoghurt

1 Preheat the oven to 200°C/400°F/Gas Mark 6. Lightly coat a baking sheet or large baking pan with vegetable oil.

2 In a large bowl, combine the vinegars, garlic, rosemary, pepper flakes, pepper and oil and whisk to mix. Add the potatoes, toss and then drain the excess marinade, saving 2 tablespoons. Spread the potatoes on the baking sheet and bake for about 45 minutes, until golden brown. It may be necessary to turn the potatoes as they bake to prevent them burning.

3 In the bowl used to toss the potatoes, combine the egg whites, onion, celery, tomato, oregano, mustard, reserved marinade and yoghurt. Toss the browned, hot potatoes with the ingredients in the bowl. Serve warm or refrigerate for at least 30 minutes to allow the flavours to come together.

Chinese noodle salad

from the Mountain Trek Fitness Retreat and Health Spa, British Columbia, Canada

Makes 4 servings

Marinade

90 ml dark sesame oil

3 tbsp balsamic vinegar

1 tbsp red pepper oil

3 tbsp chopped coriander

90 ml soy sauce

3 tbsp sugar

8-10 spring onions, thinly sliced

4 cloves garlic, minced

1 tbsp freshly ground ginger

1 x 500 g pack dried Chinese egg or rice noodles

1 Make the marinade by combining the ingredients in a bowl and stirring until the sugar has dissolved.

2 Bring a large pot of water to boil and add the noodles. Stir to prevent sticking. Cook briefly until al dente, then immediately pour the noodles into a colander and rinse with cold water.

3 Shake the colander vigorously to get rid of as much water as possible and put the noodles in a bowl.

4 Stir the marinade again, then pour half of it over the noodles and toss with your hands to distribute evenly. If the noodles aren't to be used immediately, cover with plastic wrap and refrigerate. The flavours and the heat in the red pepper will develop as the noodles stand and the noodles will keep for several days in the refrigerator.

5 Garnish with any raw vegetables finely sliced or chopped, such as red pepper, bean sprouts or mangetout. Add tofu if desired.

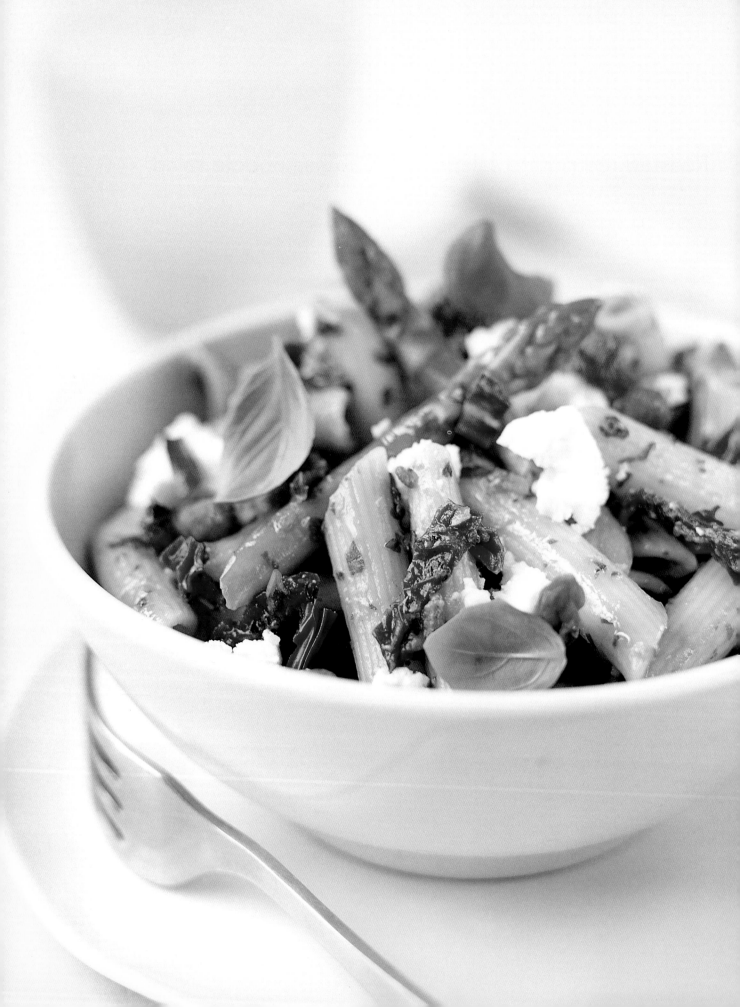

Pasta with sun-dried tomatoes and asparagus in roasted garlic-basil sauce

from Lake Austin Spa Resort, Texas, USA

Makes 4 servings

Garlic-basil sauce
2 tbsp olive oil
2 heads roasted garlic
200 g fresh basil, packed
a handful of parsley
2 tbsp Parmesan cheese
2 tbsp wine vinegar
freshly ground black pepper
pinch sugar
pinch salt
2 tbsp water

100 g sun-dried tomatoes, rehydrated, sliced
200 g blanched asparagus, cut into thirds
julienned zest of one lemon, blanched
5 cups cooked pasta
50 g feta cheese, crumbled
red pepper flakes

1 First make the garlic-basil sauce. Drizzle a drop or two of olive oil over the garlic, wrap in foil and roast at 200°C/400°F/Gas Mark 6 for 30 minutes.
2 Cool, cut the tops from the heads and squeeze out. Grind the garlic, basil and parsley in a food processor.
3 Add the remaining ingredients and process to a thin paste.
4 Rehydrate the sun-dried tomatoes in hot water for 30 minutes. Combine with the asparagus, lemon zest and pasta. Fold in the basil sauce and add the feta and red pepper.

Caesar salad

from The Golden Door Health Retreat, Queensland, Australia
Makes 4 servings

1 cos lettuce

Dressing
250 ml plain yoghurt
50 g raw cashews
3-6 cloves garlic
1-2 tbsp lemon juice
1-2 tbsp wholegrain mustard
1-2 tbsp apple juice concentrate
½ tsp sea salt

Croutons
2 cloves garlic
1 tbsp rosemary
1 tbsp olive oil
125 ml water
sea salt
100 g diced bread

1 Combine all the dressing ingredients in a blender and process until smooth. This makes about 450 ml and will keep for 2 months in the refrigerator.
2 For the croutons, blend all the ingredients, except the diced bread.
3 Toss the diced bread through the ingredients and spread on a baking tray. Bake in a hot oven until golden (approximately 10 to 15 minutes).
4 To assemble the salad, chop or tear plenty of cos lettuce and toss with the croutons and dressing.

Dinner

For most of us, our evening meal is a ritual usually associated with spending time with our partner or family or simply having time to ourselves to unwind and reflect on the day. I've selected a handful of my favourite spa recipes for this section – they may need a little more preparation time than the lunch recipes.

New guacamole

from Canyon Ranch, Arizona, USA
Makes 8 servings

50 g julienned spinach
35 g frozen peas
25 g lite silken tofu (optional)
1½ tbsp lemon juice
pinch salt
pinch cumin
pinch cayenne
pinch chilli powder
dash Tabasco sauce
6 tbsp mashed avocado
3 tbsp peeled and minced tomato
2 tbsp salsa
3 tbsp minced white onions
1 tbsp chopped cilantro
2 tsp chopped spring onions

1 Steam the spinach until wilted. Remove from the heat and squeeze out excess water.
2 Then briefly steam out any remaining excess water.
3 In a food processor, combine the spinach, peas, tofu (if desired), lemon juice, seasonings and avocado and process until smooth.
4 Fold in the remaining ingredients and mix well.

Chicken fajitas

from Canyon Ranch, Arizona, USA
Makes 4 servings

Marinade
2 tbsp low-sodium soy sauce
¼ tsp minced ginger root
¼ tsp minced garlic
2 tbsp olive oil
35 g finely chopped coriander
chilli powder
3 tbsp beer (optional)
½ tsp Tabasco sauce
½ orange, thinly sliced
½ lemon, thinly sliced
½ lime, thinly sliced
1 tbsp parsley

4 boneless chicken breast halves, skinned
100 g sliced assorted peppers
4 flour tortillas (23 cm diameter)
50 g New Guacamole (see left)
50 g salsa
125 ml fat-free sour cream

1 Combine the marinade ingredients in a shallow baking dish and mix well.
2 Cover the chicken breasts with the marinade, turning to coat evenly. Cover and refrigerate for at least 2 hours or overnight.
3 Lift the breasts from the marinade and grill for 3 to 5 minutes per side.
4 While the chicken is grilling, lightly spray a medium frying pan with non-stick vegetable oil. Over a medium heat, sauté the pepper strips until just tender. Keep warm.
5 Cut each chicken breast into strips and serve with a tortilla, some of the peppers and 2 tablespoons each of guacamole, salsa and fat-free sour cream.

Ancho chilli-dusted aubergine Parmesan with slow oven-roasted garden tomatoes

from Westward Look Resort, Arizona, USA
Makes 6 servings

6 large vine-ripe tomatoes
25 g chopped cilantro
25 g chopped parsley
3 medium aubergines
salt
freshly ground black pepper
200 g sourdough breadcrumbs
100 g grated Parmesan cheese
1 tbsp ancho chilli powder
2 eggs
125 ml milk
100 g plain flour
2 tbsp olive oil

1 Wash and core the tomatoes, then cut them in half. Place them cut side up on a baking sheet. Season with salt and freshly ground black pepper. Rub with a thin layer of olive oil and sprinkle with a quarter of the chopped herbs.
2 Place in the oven and slow roast at 130°C/250°F/Gas Mark ½ for approximately 1 hour.
3 Just before the tomatoes are ready, slice the aubergine into discs, season with salt and freshly ground black pepper and set aside. In a small mixing bowl, mix together breadcrumbs, Parmesan cheese, the rest of the chopped herbs and ancho chilli powder.
4 In another shallow bowl, scramble the eggs with the milk and set aside. To coat the aubergine, lightly dust with flour, dip in egg wash, and then coat with the breading. In a large sauté pan on medium heat, place the aubergines over the olive oil and sauté for about 3 minutes on both sides until golden.

Catch of the day with fresh herbs, lemon, garlic, mushrooms and cocktail potatoes

from the Hyatt Regency-Coolum, Queensland, Australia
Makes 4 servings

240 g peeled potatoes
200 g field mushroom
juice of 4 medium lemons
1 tsp peeled, crushed garlic
1 tsp parsley
4 tomatoes
600 g fresh fish
1 tbsp olive oil
160 g boiled brown rice
160 g baby boiled and peeled carrots
1 lemon, cut into 4 wedges
fresh herbs, to garnish

1 Roast the potatoes.
2 Steam the mushrooms whole for 6 minutes, remove from steamer and keep the remaining liquid.
3 Slice the mushrooms thinly and add to the mushroom liquid along with the lemon juice, crushed garlic and chopped herbs.
4 Cut the tomatoes in quarters, remove the seeds and cut into small pieces. Then add to the mushrooms.
5 Clean and divide the fish into four equal portions.
6 Pan-fry the fish in olive oil on both sides.
7 Cut the roasted potatoes in half and place in the frying pan together with the fish. Finish in the oven until cooked (around 8 minutes depending on the fish used).
8 Place the potatoes, boiled rice and cooked baby carrots on the bottom of the plate. Put the fish on top of the potatoes. Finish by spooning the mushroom and tomato mixture over the top and garnish with lemon and fresh herbs.

Purple basil risotto with Parmesan chips

from The Spa at Rajvilas, Jaipur, India
Makes 4 servings

50 g red peppers
50 g yellow peppers
60 g Parmesan cheese
2 tbsp olive oil
100 g shallots, chopped
2 tsp chopped garlic
200 g Arborio rice
600 ml water
125 ml white wine
60 g butter
salt
freshly ground black pepper
20 g purple basil

1 Grill and dice the peppers.
2 Grate the Parmesan cheese and put evenly on a medium hot pan, cool and remove.
3 Heat the oil and sweat the shallots and garlic. Add the Arborio rice and cook with water till just done (as described on the packet).
4 Add white wine and butter and check seasoning.
5 Purée 15 g of the basil and add to the rice together with the diced pepper.
6 Garnish with the remaining basil, shredded, and Parmesan chips.

Roasted fillets of cod with mango and tomato salsa

from Champneys, Hertfordshire, UK
Makes 4 servings

Mango and tomato salsa
1/2 mango, peeled and finely diced
1 small red onion, finely diced
2 ripe red tomatoes, skinned, deseeded and diced
2 ripe yellow tomatoes, skinned, deseeded and diced
1 garlic clove, finely chopped
1 bunch chives, chopped
1 tbsp sugar
2 tsp extra virgin olive oil
1 tbsp sherry vinegar
dash sweet chilli sauce

2 bunches asparagus
2 tbsp olive oil
4 young cod fillets (about 140 g each) scaled, skin left on and boned
800 g baby spinach or Swiss chard
salt and freshly ground pepper

1 First make the salsa. Place the mango, onion and tomatoes in a bowl, add the remaining ingredients, mix and refrigerate.
2 Heat the oven to 200°C/400°F/Gas Mark 6 and put a baking sheet in the oven to heat up.
3 Trim the asparagus into 5 cm pieces and, if necessary, trim the thick part of the stem with a peeler. Steam for 5 minutes.
4 Heat the olive oil in a non-stick frying pan. Add the fish fillets, flesh side down, and fry for 2 minutes. Place the fish skin side down on the preheated baking sheet, add the asparagus and roast in the hot oven for 7 minutes.
5 Using the same frying pan, stir-fry the spinach or chard until tender. Drain and season to taste. Place the spinach in the centre of four serving plates, pile the asparagus on top and lastly the crisp-skinned fish. Serve with the salsa.

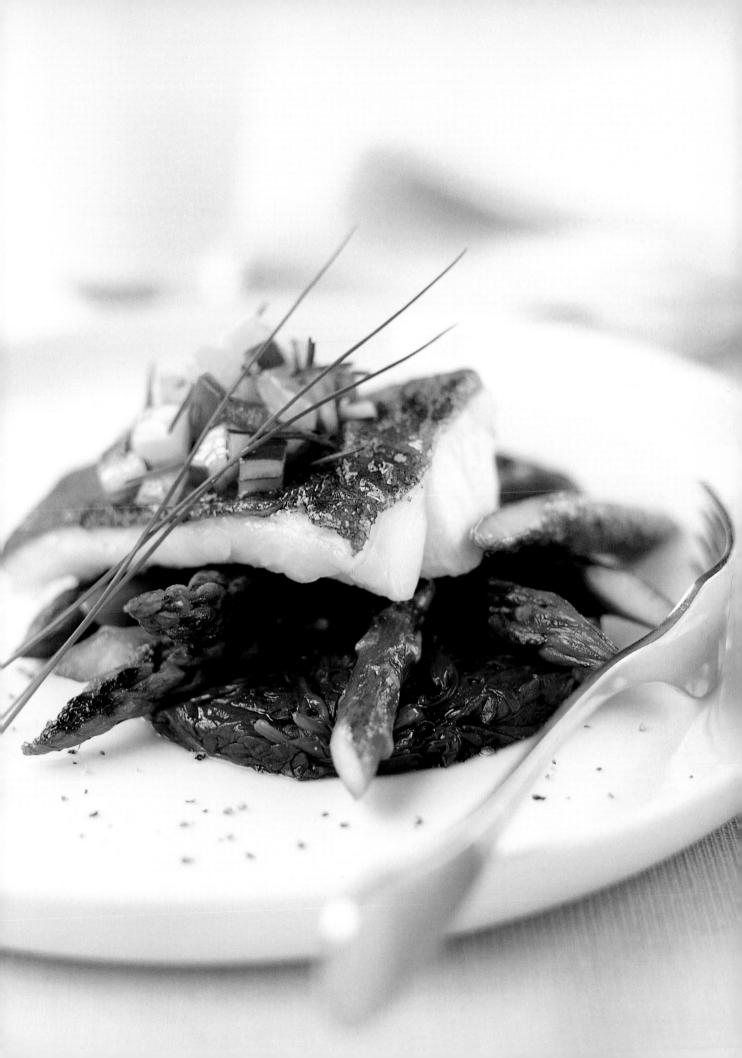

Indonesian chicken with grilled bananas

from Canyon Ranch, Arizona, USA
Makes 4 servings

Dry rub mix
½ tsp ground ginger
1 tsp ground cayenne pepper
½ tsp ground allspice
½ tsp ground cinnamon
1 tsp ground curry powder
1 tsp ground paprika
½ tsp ground turmeric
¼ tsp salt

4 skinless chicken breast halves, all fat removed
2 bananas
1 tbsp light brown sugar

1 Combine all the dry rub ingredients and mix well. Lightly coat each chicken breast with the spice mixture. Place on a plate and cover tightly. Refrigerate for at least 1 hour before grilling.
2 Pre-heat the grill. Slice the bananas into half lengthways, skins left on. Sprinkle the brown sugar on the bananas and rub it in as much as possible. Grill the bananas lightly, cut side down. Remove from the heat and set aside.
3 Remove the chicken from the refrigerator and place on the grill. Grill for about 5 minutes on each side until done.
4 Serve each grilled chicken breast with a grilled banana half still in the peel.

Grilled garden vegetable platter

from Westward Look Resort, Arizona, USA
Makes 8 servings

1 bunch of Italian parsley
1 tbsp fresh thyme leaves
3 cloves of garlic, freshly chopped
1 tbsp crushed red pepper flakes
freshly ground black pepper to taste
450 ml olive oil
2 medium courgettes
2 medium yellow squash
4 medium tomatoes
2 green chillis
2 red peppers
salt

1 Rinse the parsley, pat dry and then finely chop.
2 Pick the fresh thyme leaves from the stems. In a bowl, add the parsley and thyme together with the garlic, red pepper flakes, freshly ground black pepper and olive oil.
3 Slice the vegetables into 12 mm-thick long slices. Toss the vegetables with enough marinade to coat lightly. Let them chill in the refrigerator for about an hour.
4 Remove the vegetables from the bowl and place flat on a baking sheet pan and season to taste with salt and freshly ground black pepper.
5 Transfer the vegetables and grill over a high heat for approximately 1½ minutes on each side, or until desired crispness.
6 Place back on the rinsed baking sheet to chill to room temperature. Serve as appetisers.

Smooth delights

We all like the occasional treat, but all too often it's in the form of a fat and calorie packed packet of crisps or chocolate bar. There's nothing wrong with having the odd indulgence but if you are trying to re-educate your palette and detox your system, why not try some of the health-conscious treats on offer at the world's leading health spas and resorts.

Banana, citrus and oat smoothie

from Champneys, Hertfordshire, UK
Makes 4 servings

50 g rolled oats
100 ml skimmed milk
3 small bananas
finely grated zest and juice of 1 orange
finely grated zest and juice of 1 lemon
150 ml low-fat yoghurt
150 ml low-fat fromage frais
3 tbsp clear honey
pinch mixed spice
8 ice cubes

1 Put the oats in a bowl, add the milk and leave to soak overnight in the refrigerator.
2 Keep the fruit, yoghurt and fromage frais in the refrigerator overnight.
3 In the morning, chop the bananas and place in a blender with all the remaining ingredients. Blend until smooth, then pass through a fine sieve and serve in iced glasses with more ice and straws.

Banana smoothie

from Lucknam Park, Wiltshire, UK
Makes 1 serving

200 g bananas
175 ml semi-skimmed milk
1 tbsp natural yoghurt
2 tbsp clear honey
40 g vanilla ice cream
4 ice cubes

1 Combine all the ingredients in a food processor and blend until smooth. Serve in a chilled glass.

Paradise punch

from Canyon Ranch, Arizona, USA
Makes 1 serving

125 ml skimmed milk
125 ml unsweetened pineapple juice
2 tbsp non-fat cottage cheese
½ tsp sugar
¼ tsp vanilla extract
¼ tsp coconut extract
2 ice cubes

1 Combine all the ingredients in a food processor and blend until smooth. Serve in a chilled glass.

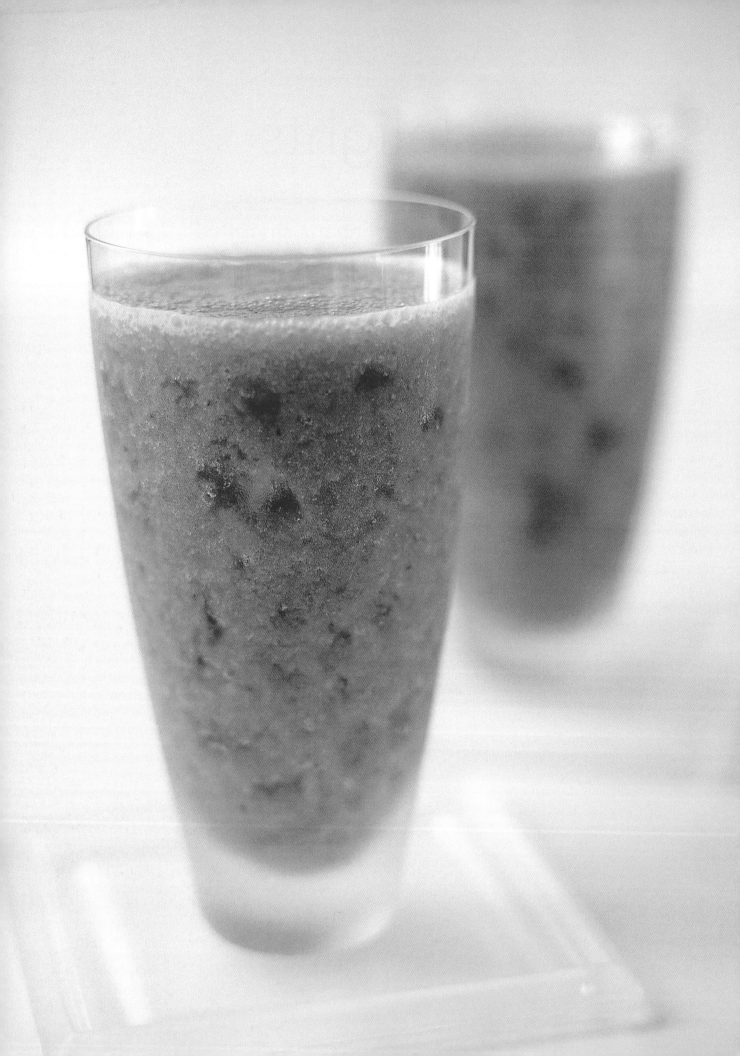

Strawberry-banana smoothie

from Rancho La Puerta, Baja California, Mexico

Makes 2 servings

400 g hulled strawberries
2 bananas
250 ml unsweetened, unfiltered apple juice
2 to 3 tbsp fresh lime juice
ice cubes
mint leaves to garnish (optional)

1 Combine all the ingredients in a food processor and blend until smooth. Pour into glasses with mint leaves on top, if using, and serve immediately.

Energiser smoothie

from the Golden Door, California, USA

Makes 2 servings

175 ml fresh orange juice
175 ml low-fat plain yoghurt
1 banana
4 to 5 pitted dates, cut into pieces
1 tbsp wheat or oat germ

1 Put all the ingredients into a blender and process until smooth and creamy.
2 Serve immediately.

Original Golden Door potassium broth

from the Golden Door, California, USA

Makes 12 servings

This is one of my all-time favourite brews, reminding me of my first trip to the Golden Door spa and my morning hike up the mountain. As Michel Stroot, executive chef at the spa, explains, Potassium Broth is incredibly replenishing if you've been exercising and as an energy boost. 'Potassium, available in fruits and vegetables, is an important mineral that needs replenishing after an energetic workout, when it is lost [as much as 500 to 600 milligrams after two or three hours of strenuous exercise]. This is why we serve this mid-morning by the pool after our guests have hiked, weight-trained and participated in aerobics classes. They need it! And they love it.'

12 to 14 plum tomatoes, quartered, or 1 x 800 g can crushed plum tomatoes
400 g chopped vegetable trimmings, such as celery stalks and leaves, onions, carrots, cabbage, peppers and parsley stems
2 garlic cloves, crushed
1 tbsp dried basil or chopped fresh basil leaves
1 tsp red pepper flakes (optional)

1 In a large saucepan, combine the tomatoes, vegetable trimmings, garlic, basil, pepper flakes (if using) and 2.5 litres of water and bring to the boil over a high heat. Reduce the heat and simmer, uncovered, for about 45 minutes until the flavours blend.
2 Strain the broth through a sieve, gently pressing on the solids to extract as much flavour as possible. Discard the solids. Serve hot.

Desserts

The idea that health spas and desserts do not go together is, quite frankly, a myth. Providing that you stick to moderate portions and don't go overboard, a dessert is the ideal way to complete a meal. I've gathered my personal favourites from a host of mouth-watering temptations from the top ranking spas across the globe. Naturally, they are only a taster of what you will find at a spa but they do make you realise that you can have something sweet.

Strawberry cheesecake

from Henlow Grange Health Farm, Bedfordshire, UK
Makes 4 servings

75 g muesli
125 ml apple juice
2 tsp plain flour
125 ml strawberry purée
100 ml natural yoghurt
100 ml low-fat cream cheese
4 tsp gelatine powder
2 tsp sweetener
1 punnet strawberries

1 Line four ramekins with greaseproof paper. Mix the muesli, apple juice and flour and press into the ramekins.
2 Combine the purée, cream cheese, natural yoghurt and sweetener and set with the gelatine.
3 Pour into the ramekins and refrigerate.
4 Serve decorated with fresh strawberries.

Carrot cake

from Canyon Ranch, Arizona, USA
Makes 24 servings

300 g wholewheat flour
1½ tsp baking powder
1½ tsp cinnamon
pinch salt
4 egg yolks
5 tbsp sunflower oil
60 ml buttermilk
60 ml fructose
1½ tsp vanilla essence
60 g chopped walnuts, toasted
300 g grated carrots
1¾ crushed pineapple, drained
6 egg whites
60 ml fructose
pinch baking powder
1½ tsp corn oil margarine
1½ tsp corn syrup
6 tbsp buttermilk
1½ tsp vanilla essence

1 Preheat the oven to 170°C/325°F/Gas Mark 3. Spray a 23 x 33 cm pan with non-stick vegetable coating. Sift the flour, baking powder, cinnamon and salt into a deep bowl.
2 In a medium bowl, combine the egg yolks, oil, buttermilk, fructose and vanilla. Add to the flour mixture and stir in until combined. Stir in the walnuts, carrots and pineapple.
3 In a small bowl, beat the egg whites until they hold a peak. Fold into the batter. Pour the mixture into the pan and bake for 30 to 35 minutes. The cake is done when it springs back when pushed in the centre. Remove from the oven and cool slightly.
4 For the glaze, combine the remaining ingredients, except the vanilla, in a saucepan and bring to the boil. Reduce the heat and simmer for 5 minutes. Remove the glaze from heat and stir in the vanilla. Use a fork to poke holes in the top of the cake. Pour the glaze over the warm cake.

Filo pastry apple strudel

from the Golden Door, California, USA

Makes 6 servings

This is simply the best apple strudel I've ever tasted and even more pleasure was derived from it by learning to make it in none other than the kitchen of The Golden Door itself. Part of the spa's programme includes an evening cookery class where you can learn some of the spa's best-loved recipes so that you can take home a little piece for yourself – literally. Even if you're not a big dessert fan, don't miss this one.

5 Golden Delicious apples, peeled, cored and sliced
2 tsp ground cinnamon
pinch ground cloves
25 g raisins or dried cranberries
75 g brown sugar
five 30 x 43 cm sheets of filo pastry
icing sugar for sprinkling

1 Coat a large non-stick sauté pan with vegetable oil spray and sauté the apples with the cinnamon, cloves, raisins and brown sugar over a medium heat for 8 to 10 minutes, stirring frequently, until the apples begin to soften. Transfer to a bowl to cool.

2 Preheat the oven to 180°C/350°F/Gas Mark 4. Spray a baking sheet with vegetable oil spray.

3 Place 1 sheet of the filo pastry on a work surface with a long side towards you and spray it with vegetable oil spray. Stack the remaining filo sheets on top, spraying each sheet. Spoon the apple filling in a long row across the centre of the dough. Starting with the long side facing you, roll up the dough around the filling to enclose it. Tuck in the ends and transfer to the baking sheet, seam side down.

4 Lightly spray the top of the roll with vegetable oil spray. Bake for 35 to 40 minutes, until the pastry is golden brown. Sprinkle with icing sugar, cut into slices and serve warm.

Berry compote

from The Greenhouse, Texas, USA

Makes 12 servings

225 g fresh raspberries
175 g fresh blueberries
225 g fresh strawberries cut into quarters
2 tbsp orange zest
100 g raspberries, fresh or frozen
2 tbsp sugar-free strawberry fruit spread
½ banana, peeled

1 Place the fresh raspberries, blueberries, strawberries and orange zest into a bowl.

2 Place the fresh or frozen raspberries, the fruit spread and banana into a food processor and blend until smooth. Strain the mixture if desired.

3 Add the puréed mixture into the berries and orange zest mixture and toss gently. Keep refrigerated.

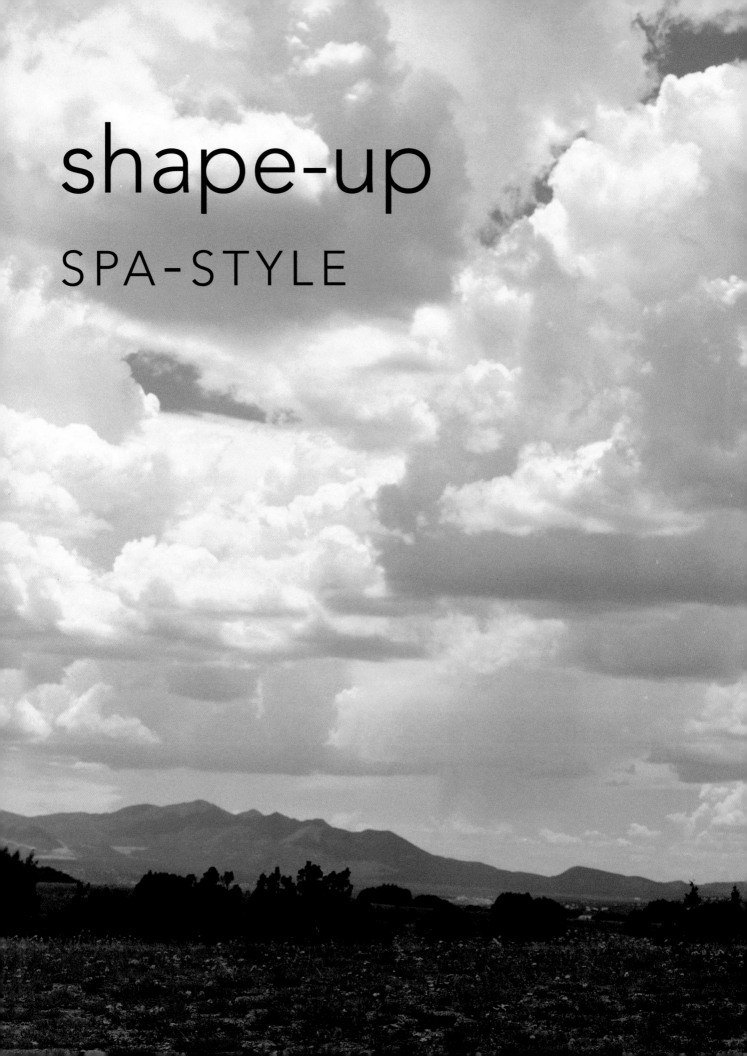

shape-up
SPA-STYLE

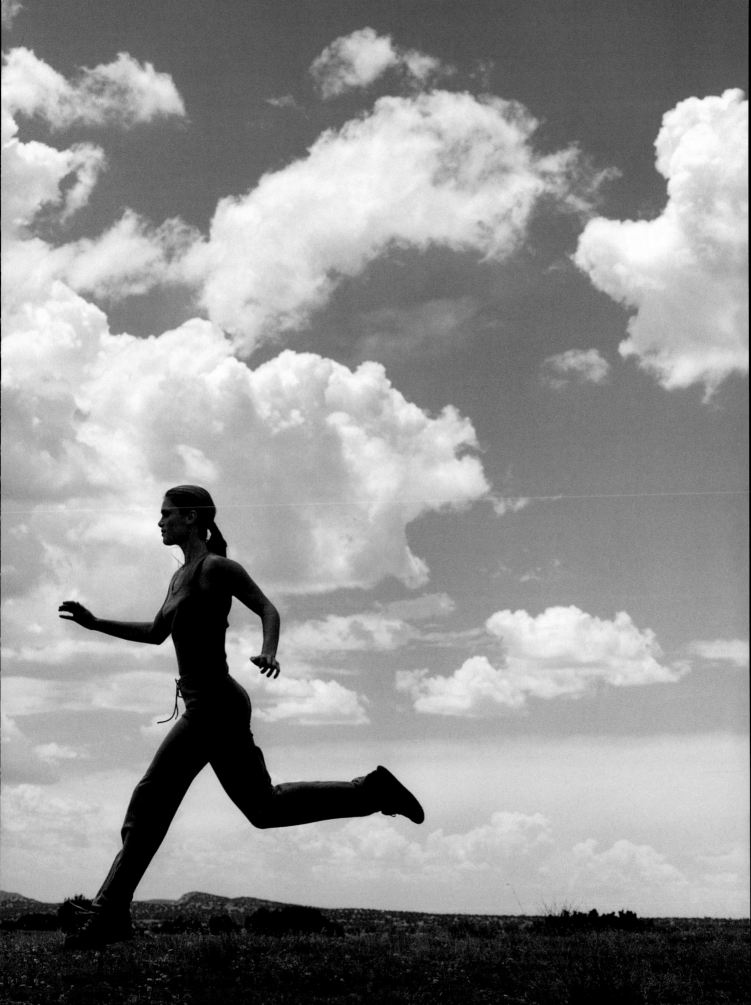

Time to get going

Part of the pleasure of checking into a spa is the knowledge that, with a little bit of effort, you can check out a week later not only looking better but feeling healthier and actually being fitter. A spa break is often the vital kick-start that we need to motivate us from a passive state to an active one. Let's be honest. It's all too easy to become a couch potato at home when you expend so much of your energy at work, and leisure time just doesn't seem to have a place in your busy never-rest-for-a-minute lifestyle. While a spa break may not fit into your non-stop schedule at this moment, you can benefit from the fitness expertise available at the world's top spas.

Going to the gym is often the last thing any of us wants to do at the end of a frenetic day and even though we know it does us good, we just don't seem to have the right motivation. The solution? We've asked the experts from the international spas, the Golden Door, California, USA; Echo Valley Ranch, Jesmond, Canada, and St David's Hotel, Cardiff; Henlow Grange Health Farm, Bedfordshire and Ragdale Hall Health Hydro, Leicestershire, UK, to share their fitness secrets, motivation tricks and get-you-back-in-shape moves so you can get on track. From walking to weight training, spa fitness experts give their advice on activities that you can do easily at home. And to increase your flexibility, there are stretching exercises to tone your muscles.

From boosting your immune system to relieving stress and reducing depression, there are a million good reasons to exercise. A recent government report suggested that even 30 minutes of physical activity each day would lead to significant improvements in health and well being. These include a reduction in the risk of developing heart disease, stroke, non-insulin dependent diabetes and hip fractures due to osteoporosis. In addition, exercise improves brain function, helps to lower blood cholesterol and blood pressure levels and promote sounder sleep.

CREATE YOUR OWN EXERCISE PROGRAMME

An effective exercise programme, according to the experts at The Spa at St David's Hotel needs to promote aerobic endurance, flexibility and strength. Thankfully, aerobic endurance exercise doesn't mean that you need to run a marathon. You can change aspects of your lifestyle to fit aerobic endurance into your life as well as setting aside time for training. For example, instead of getting the bus or tube to work, cycle or walk or, if walking the whole way isn't an option, get off the bus or train a few stops early and walk the rest of the way. Even small sacrifices, like walking up and down the stairs instead of taking the lift every day, will help.

One of the biggest hurdles to get over is actually motivating yourself to begin and then stick to an exercise programme. So, here, Dean L. Hodgkin, BSc PEA Cert, a global Reebok trainer and consultant to Ragdale Hall Health Hydro, shares his motivational tips, guaranteed to get you off the couch, once and for all.

1 FOCUS

It is time to move but so often thinking about doing it is what is difficult. It is always easier once you get going. (Ever had a day when the journey to the gym was harder than the workout?) So make a start as soon as possible.

Commit yourself to improving with every fibre of your being and you will be amazed at how many hurdles you can overcome. If you are not really committed, you might as well give up, as you are unlikely to see great results.

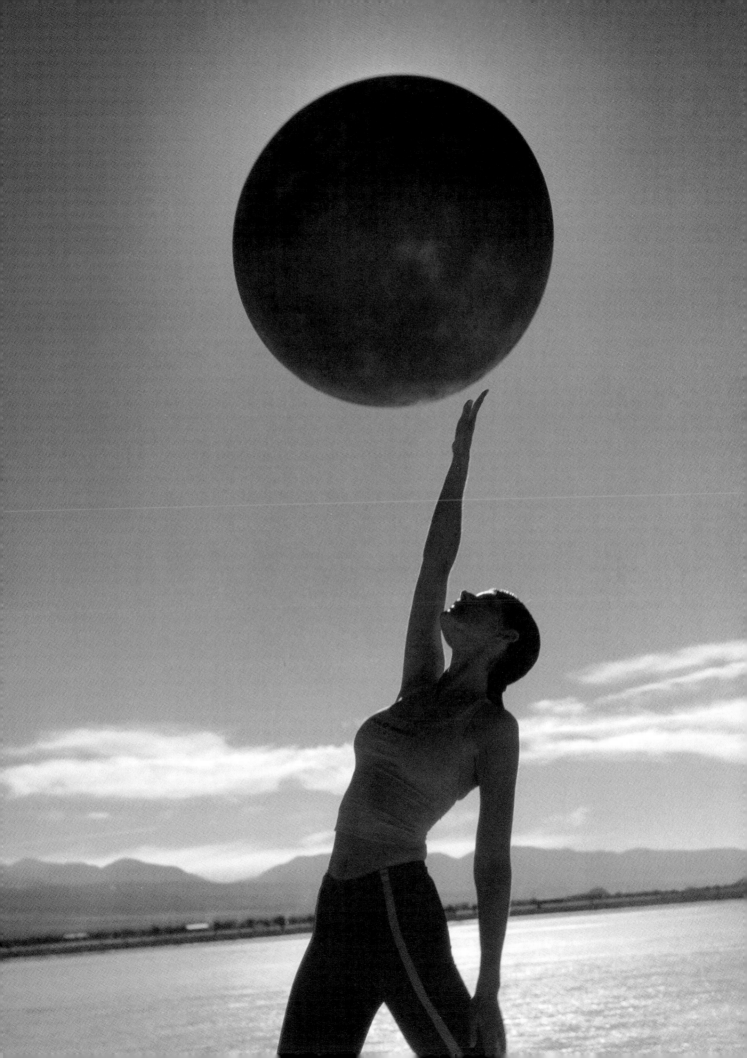

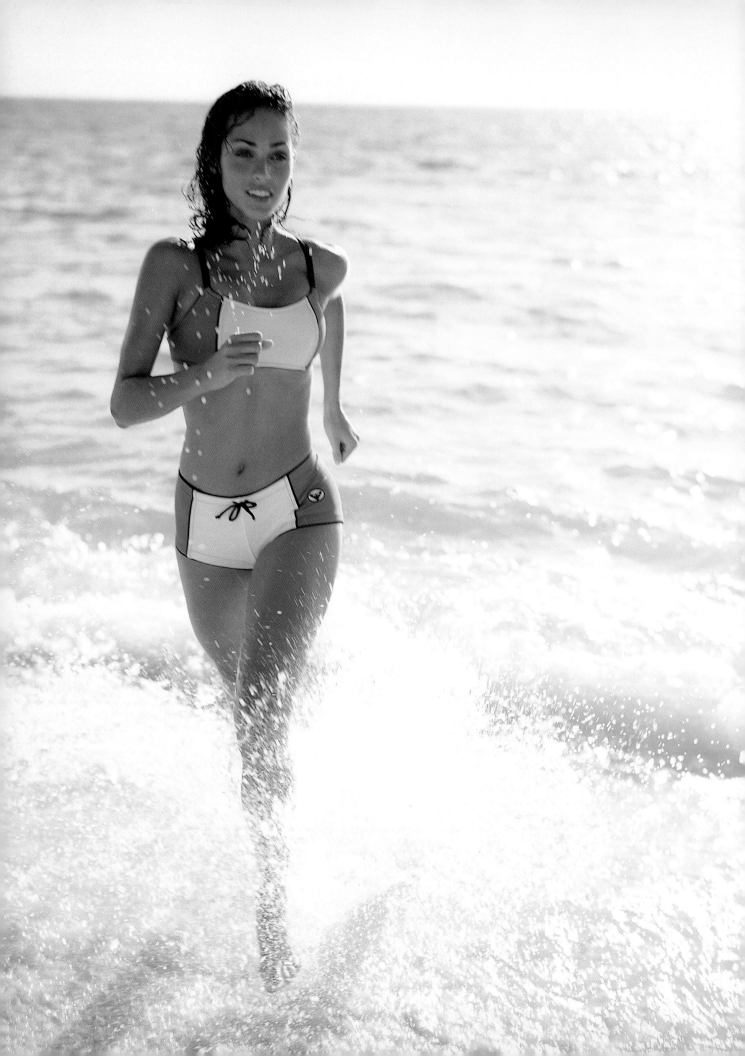

2 THINK POSITIVE

From the outside, life will always present obstacles, which have to be worked around, under, over or through if you are truly committed to getting fitter. But it is all too easy to sabotage progress from the inside with that small voice that says, 'You'll never make it', or the perverse part of our nature that holds us back from doing whatever it takes to move on. Look to beat this self-defeating behaviour by replacing it with more constructive thought patterns. Think positive and you are far more likely to achieve what you set out to do.

If you feel overwhelmed by the enormity of your task, remember that before you know it small steps will add up to big steps. Take one step at a time and congratulate yourself after every one. Your prize awaits you. To help set yourself some goals see right, and then check regularly that what you are doing is taking you closer to reaching them. If it is not, you need to adapt your goals, which of course is fine. Try something daily towards reaching your goals, don't leave it until tomorrow.

Zap any negative thoughts with the power of positive thinking. Tell yourself daily that you will achieve your goal, visualise yourself winning through any adversity and enjoying the rewards your goals will bring you.

Spend time with positive people too (not everyone will agree that goals are possible or be happy that you are changing). Friends that support you and colleagues that motivate you will prove invaluable in your desire to move on up. Sharing your workouts with someone can be fun and you can inspire each other to keep going.

Talking of other people, if you know someone who has already achieved what you are setting out to do, decide if what worked for them will work for you. By adopting their habits you may save yourself time – they will have taken some of the trial and error out for you!

It may also help you to move forwards if you remember how you achieved other difficult things in the past, but that you did what it took and you got there in the end.

3 LIVE AND LEARN

There will still be times when things do not go according to plan and you do not move on as much as you would like. If you have lost your focus go back and look at your goals. Thinking about how much you will enjoy achieving them will put you back in the game again. If it's a mistake that is getting you down, try thinking of it simply as a result you created through a certain action. If you change the action you will create a new result.

SETTING GOALS

If you are not exactly sure what you want, spend some time asking yourself these questions:
• What would you do if you knew you couldn't fail?
• What do you love doing?
• What skills do you already have that when you use them you are successful?
• What will the year ahead be like if you don't take the next step?
• Once you have decided on your goal, or goals, write them down (yes, committing them to paper really does seem to help!). Then set yourself a realistic time frame for each goal and decide how to start moving towards them.
• Be specific – if you are not sure where you are going, you may not like where you end up! Exactly what do you want to achieve? What will this feel like? What difference will this make to your life?

Mix and match

No two bodies are the same so the chances are that an exercise programme that is right for someone else may not work for you. The secret to sticking to an exercise regime is to find one that's personalised to you. It goes without saying that a trip to a spa or going to the gym regularly will give you a head start. A qualified fitness instructor can help you to work out a schedule that suits your lifestyle. But the good news is that you can get on to the right track yourself by following a few golden rules. Fitness expert, Julie Pelletier, from Echo Valley Ranch Resort, Jesmond, Canada shares her tips and training know-how.

One of the most common mistakes that we make when we begin an exercise programme is to exercise too much. At the beginning, we tend to be very motivated and exercise four times and more a week when for years that's what we've been doing in a whole year. So in terms of long-term motivation, start very slowly, maybe working out twice a week, and not more, even if you want to. If you can maintain this over a one-month period, then add one workout per week. It is far better to exercise twice a week for an extended period than to exercise six times a week for three weeks and then stop because of lack of motivation or injury. People can't expect to go from zero workouts per week to playing tennis or jogging four times a week without suffering injuries. The body has to be able to adapt. And it doesn't happen overnight.

Another common situation that causes a decrease in interest is the fact that people often do the same workout over and over again. That's where a technique called Cross Training comes into play, which involves doing a variety of physical activities. On Monday, go to a park for a walk. On Wednesday, do home weight training. On Thursday, go cycling. And on Saturday, try a jog-walk mix (see Cross Training ideas overleaf). In this way, you avoid doing the same thing all the time. By being active in various ways, the risk of getting injured diminishes and multiple muscles are being used. And in this way, if on Monday it's raining, you can switch to an indoor weight training session. Or if you don't feel like biking on Wednesday, you can take a walk instead. Do what you feel like doing.

Instead of going to the gym on Saturday morning, why not go ice-skating on Saturday night or find a local boat club and try a bit of kayaking. If it's too hot and humid to go for a jog, go to a local pool and do your jogging programme in the pool, in either deep or shallow water.

ACTIVITY GUIDE

Want to find the activity best suited to your fitness requirements? Fitness expert, Dean L. Hodgkin, gives the low-down on the top spa fitness activities that are also suitable for at-home or health club practice. We have then taken the first three suggestions – stretching, weight training and walking – and provided you with programmes on pages 78-83 to get you underway.

Strengthening stretches (see pages 78-9): doing strengthening stretches for 10 minutes twice a week is not much, but it is much better than nothing. You could also include some exercises during a walk: when you pass some steps, do some heel raises; when you pass a tree, do push-ups against it, and when you pass a bench, do step-ups. Finish with abdominal exercises at home and more stretching.

Weight training (see pages 80-1): this is the best form of exercise to change your body shape and it will speed up your metabolic rate, meaning your body will burn up more calories, even while you sleep. It is important to get a trainer to teach you safe techniques and to ensure the programme is balanced, so reducing any risk of injury. A huge plus is the bone strengthening that occurs, thus reducing a risk of osteoporosis.

KICK-START YOURSELF

Here's an example of a kick-start fitness programme to take you from couch potato to regular exerciser. Begin by committing to working out twice a week.
• 15 minutes of aerobic exercise such as walking or cycling.
• 10 minutes strengthening stretches.
Then you should feel able to take on more strenuous forms of exercise on a regular basis. Just take that initial step and you will soon find yourself getting into the swing of things.

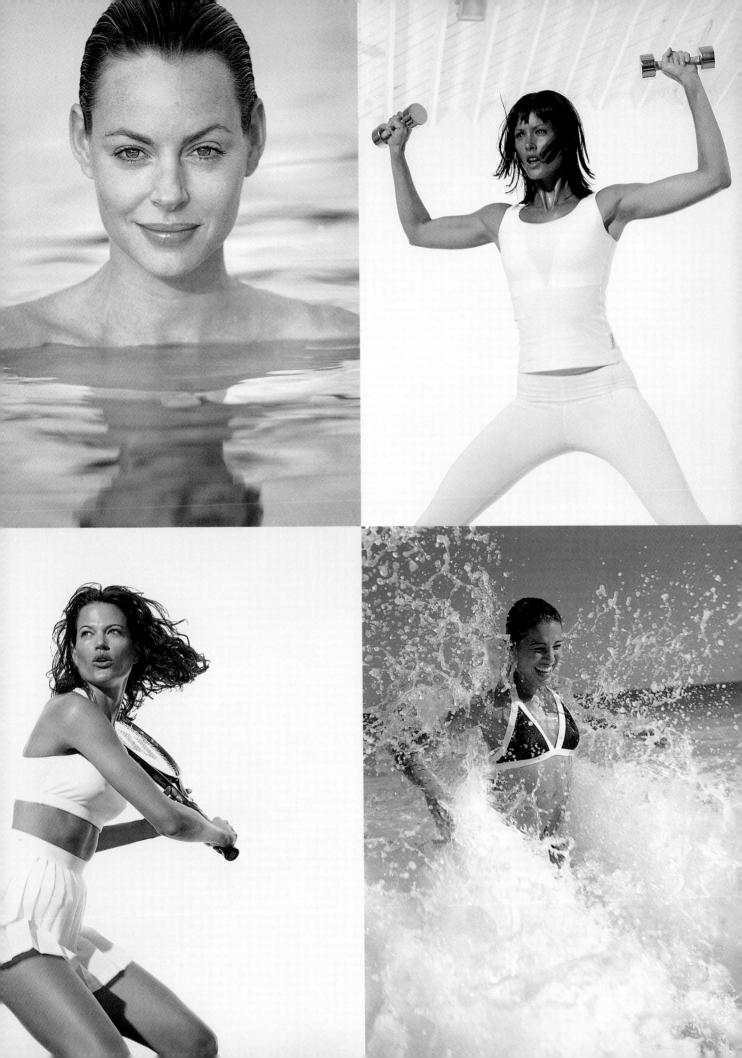

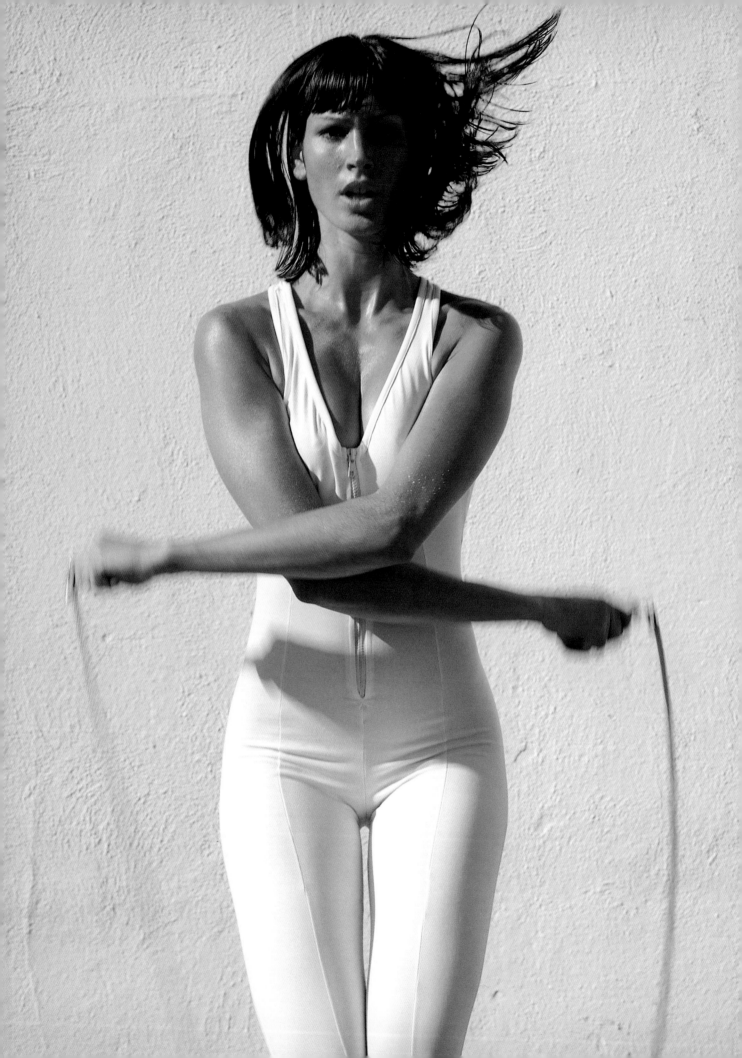

Power walking (see pages 82-3): this is a fantastic way of getting fit because it is so accessible, whatever your age or fitness level. A great component in weight-loss programmes, power walking has been shown to have considerable stress-reducing properties related to the endorphin 'high', which is more pronounced when exercise is taken outdoors. It is a great choice for anyone who is overweight as the stress in the joints is reduced but you can still achieve a suitable intensity level via varying the pace in intervals or perhaps introducing inclines.

Swimming: a triple whammy, as this is a good calorie consumer, improves the efficiency of the heart and lungs and helps to tone the whole body due to the resistive properties of the exercise medium – water. The best thing about this activity is that due to the cooling and comforting effects of the water, you tend not to feel as if you are working as hard as in the gym or a class. To get the best out of it, forget the breaststroke and go for the crawl.

Canoeing: helps prevent lower back trouble by forcing you to use your core (trunk) strength muscle, due to sitting upright with legs out in front. The shoulders, arms and upper back will get a magnificent toning effect, so pull the shoulder pads out of all those eighties' power suits.

Cycling: while studio cycling is now very popular, opt for getting out and about as there are noticeable mood improvements from changing scenery and the interaction with nature. It has good potential for calorific expenditure but toning effects are limited to the lower body and an overuse may lead to kyphotic (round shoulders) characteristics, so balance this with a good post-exercise stretch.

Tennis: not too useful in weight loss as there is a lot of stop and start, but can be a great way to vent aggression in a harmless way. Super toning effects for the legs but over time can take its toll on the hips, knees and ankles. Since it is a unilateral activity, other sessions will be required to balance stresses in the musculoskeletal system.

CROSS TRAINING

To vary your workout, try some of the following ideas:

Jog/walk mix or walk/skip mix: jogging improves aerobic fitness but as it is high impact, it can place stress on the joints. So ensure that you have a very good pair of shoes with ample shock absorption. Jogging provides great toning for the lower body and is an excellent calorie burner but use it in tandem with other exercises to achieve all-round improvements. Here's how.
Do a mix of jogging and walking. Example: for a beginner, walk 5 minutes as a warm-up. Then jog 2 minutes and walk 3 minutes and repeat 4 times, then 10 minutes normal walking. Or any other pattern would be fine. If you want to increase the jogging portion, you could move to 2 minutes of jogging and 2 minutes of walking. Work up to getting a full 20 minutes of jogging.
Think safely – do not run alone at night in areas that are not well lit.

Give it some rope: skipping is a very good cardiovascular exercise, but in reality, who wants to be skipping for 20 minutes – or who can? One way to integrate skipping into a workout could be to go for a 30 minutes walk and include four periods of skipping into it. It would increase the intensity of the walk, and probably make it more challenging: try skipping for 1 minute without mistakes, try beating your own record, or skipping without mistake longer than your friend.

Take the stairs: another idea to increase the intensity of a walk and work on your thighs and buttock muscles would be to do 'stairs' – if your park or gym has some. Go up and down the stairs a few times. If you are agile enough, take two stairs at a time. Very good for strengthening the legs.

Stretch and strengthen

Stretching is a very important aspect of a fitness programme to maintain flexibility, particularly as we age. When given proper stretching exercises, people with lower back, neck, elbow or knee problems can find the pain diminishes. A study found that 80 percent of people would have back pain at one point during their lives. So as a preventive tool or as part of a treatment, stretching can be used. The best way to learn proper technique would be to consult an exercise specialist, such as an athletic therapist, sports physiotherapist. Then you can do it on your own. A lot of exercises can be done at work while sitting in front of a computer or while watching television.

GUIDELINES
• Warm up for at least 5 minutes before you begin with light cardiovascular activities, such as walking or cycling.
• Exercise on a firm, padded surface. Place a small pillow or folded towel under the head and neck when lying on your back or under your hips and forehead when lying face down.
• During stretch exercises, breathe normally. Move into each position slowly and stretch only to the point of mild tension – no pain. Hold the stretch without bouncing or straining. Stretching can be done daily, or at least every other day.
• Perform each strength and stabilisation exercise at a slow pace to the point of moderate muscle fatigue. Breathe normally or exhale on the exertion phase of each exercise. Start with a few repetitions and gradually increase to 10-15 if possible. Stabilisation and strength exercises should be done every other day for best results.
• During stabilisation exercises, contract your abdominal muscles to maintain a neutral position of the pelvis. Keep the shoulders gently pulled back and down while keeping the nape of the neck long and the chin level.
• Avoid or modify the exercises that cause pain by decreasing the range of motion and/or the number of repetitions.
• In addition to performing this programme regularly, it is important to participate in low or non-impact cardiovascular activities such as walking, cycling or swimming.

The spa stretching regime
from the Golden Door, California, USA

The following stretches have been designed by the fitness experts at The Golden Door. Not only will they help to lengthen and strengthen muscles, they are also designed to strengthen and increase the flexibility of the muscles of the spine and to improve posture.

THE EXERCISES
Stretch: lower back
Lie on your back with your knees bent directly over your waistline. Hold behind the thighs and bring your knees towards your chest. The knees can be together or slightly apart. Hold for 15 to 30 seconds. Repeat 1 to 2 times.

Stretch: hip flexor
Lie on your back, place your hands behind one thigh and pull towards your chest. Rotate each ankle 5 times in each direction. Keep the other leg straight and press the calf towards the floor. Hold for 15 to 30 seconds. Repeat 1 to 2 times.

Stretch: hip and buttocks
Lie on your back with your left foot on the floor and right ankle crossed over the left thigh. Press the right knee away from your body. Lift the left foot off the floor and bring the left thigh towards your chest. Reach through your legs and hold on to the back of the left thigh (a). Repeat on the other side. Hold for 15 to 30 seconds. Repeat 1 to 2 times each leg.

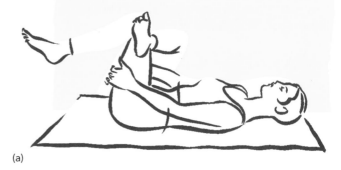

(a)

Stretch: side lying quad

Lie on one side with your head cradled in your bottom arm and with the bottom leg slightly bent. Hold on to the top ankle and pull towards your buttocks while pressing your hips forwards and keeping your leg parallel to the floor (b). Repeat on other leg. Hold for 15 to 30 seconds. Repeat 1 to 2 times.

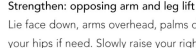

(b)

Stabilisation: bridging

With your feet a hip-width apart and knees bent at 90 degrees, slowly raise your buttocks from the floor, keeping your abdominals tight and hips even. Lower one vertebra at a time. Repeat 5 to 10 times.

Stretch: abdominal curl

Lie on your back with your legs up on a chair (or with your knees bent and feet on the floor) and with your hands behind your head or across your chest. While keeping your head aligned with your spine, tighten your abdominals by lifting the shoulders off the floor (c). Repeat 5 to 10 times.

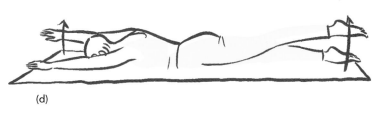

(c)

Strengthen: opposing arm and leg lift

Lie face down, arms overhead, palms down. Use a towel under your hips if need. Slowly raise your right arm and left leg, without twisting your hips or shoulders (d). Exhale. Return to the starting position and then work on the alternate sides. Pull in your abdominals and keep your neck and shoulders relaxed. Hold for 3 to 5 seconds. Repeat 10 to 15 times.

(d)

Strengthen: wall squat

With your head, shoulders and hips against a wall, walk your feet away from the wall about 60 to 90 cm. Position your feet a hip-width apart, bend your knees to 45 degrees (work up to 90 degrees). Keep your knees aligned over your ankles, lift your toes off the floor and hold the position. Hold for 20 to 60 seconds. Repeat 3 to 5 times.

Stretch: lower back and abdominals

Lie on your stomach with your legs straight and forearms and chest on the floor. Press up your torso while keeping your hips flat on the floor, head square and eyes looking forwards (e). Hold for 5 seconds. Then return to the start. Repeat 3 to 5 times.

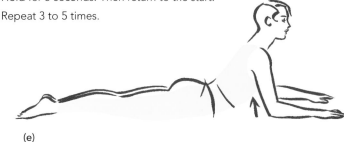

(e)

Hand weight training

There is a very good reason to incorporate weight training into your fitness routine. After the age of 25, you lose about half a pound of muscle every year. Worse still, if you don't exercise, fat replaces muscle. Not only does your shape begin to suffer, but your strength decreases too. Add to this the fact that, as we age, the risk of osteoporosis (brittle bone disease) increases and the picture is not looking good. Working out with weights, however, goes some way towards protecting against muscle loss and decreased bone density.

GUIDELINES

• Perform each exercise at a slow, controlled pace, on two to three non-consecutive days per week.
• Exhale on the difficult (exertion) part of the exercise, or breathe normally.
• Exercises for one of the large muscle groups (leg, back, and chest) should be performed before the smaller muscle groups (arms, calves).
• Follow the programme in the order outlined.
• Complete the exercises for each muscle group before moving on to the next.
• Increase repetitions, weight and/or sets gradually for continuous improvements. For general strength training, increase to next weight when you reach 12 repetitions comfortably. Use a chart to show your progression.
• Rest for 30/45 seconds between sets if using heavy weights (3.6 kg or more for women, 5.4 kg or more for men). For lighter weights, rest 20 to 30 seconds between sets.
• For all standing upper body exercises, stand with feet comfortably apart, knees relaxed and hips tucked under.
• Perform each exercise through the full range of motion without snapping joints. Never compromise sound technique or good posture to finish a repetition.

The spa hand weight-training programme
from Henlow Grange Health Farm, Bedfordshire, UK

WARM-UP EXERCISES

1 Warm-up on a bike treadmill or do any other rhythmical activity for at least 5 minutes.
2 Do shoulder rolls. Stand or sit with arms down at the sides. Circle shoulders forwards 5 times and back 5 times.
3 Do arm circles. Perform slow, large arm circles with elbows slightly bent. Perform 5 forward and 5 back.
4 Do sky reaches. Stand with feet apart, knees relaxed and pelvis tilted up. With arms overhead, reach alternate hands towards the ceiling, bending slightly at the waist. Perform 5 each side.
5 Do squats. With feet 100-120 cm apart and toes slightly turned out, slowly bend knees halfway, keeping heels flat on the floor and knees aligned over the ankles, then straighten. Perform 5 to 10 times.
6 Stretch out the muscles that are going to be used, holding each stretch for 8 to 10 seconds.

WEIGHT TRAINING EXERCISES

Legs: squats
Stand with your feet a hip-width apart, toes forwards, arms straight at sides, hands grasping weights. Bend your legs halfway, keeping your back straight. Flexing at the hips, lean forwards slightly and imagine that you are sitting in a chair with heels down.

Legs: heel raises
Stand with your feet slightly apart, with your arms straight at your sides and hands grasping the weights. Perform the exercise from the following three foot positions: toes forwards, toes out, toes in. Keeping your legs straight, lift your heels off the floor. Rise on to your toes then lower your heels.

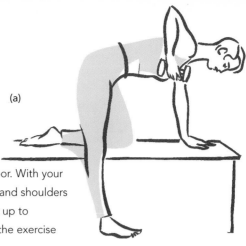

(a)

Back: single arm row

Place your left hand and left knee on a bench and keep your right foot on the floor. With your right arm straight, grasp a weight in your right hand. Keeping your back straight and shoulders square, bend your right elbow, aiming it towards the ceiling, bringing the weight up to underarm and squeezing the shoulder blade (a). Do not twist your back. Repeat the exercise with the other arm.

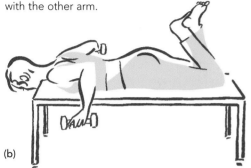

(b)

Back: reverse flies

Lie face down on a bench, elbows slightly bent. Grasp the weights below the bench, palms facing inwards. Lift the weights out to the sides at shoulder level while squeezing your shoulder blades together (b).

Chest: bench press

Lie back on a bench, knees bent, feet flat on bench and elbows bent at shoulder level. Grasp the weights at shoulder height, palms facing knees. Keeping your arms a shoulder-width apart, press the weights towards the ceiling and straighten your arms above your chest (d). Avoid locking out the elbows.

(d)

Shoulders: shoulder press

Sit or stand upright with your legs apart. Grasp the weights above your shoulders with palms facing forwards. Bend your elbows, points outwards. Press the weights over your head in a straight line alongside your ears.

Shoulders: upright row

Stand with your legs apart. Grasp the weights in front of your thighs with your palms facing the thighs. Bend your elbows while lifting the weights to your chin. Attempt to lift your elbows higher than the weights.

Triceps: tricep kick back

Stand or sit upright with your elbows pulled backwards at your sides. Grasp the weights next to your chest, palms facing each other. Straighten your arms, pushing the weights back (c). Keep your elbows pulled into your sides.

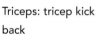

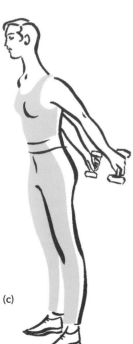

(c)

Biceps: pull-ups

Stand or sit upright with your elbows pulled into your sides. Grasp the weights in front of your thighs with your palms facing forwards. Keeping your elbows at your side, bend your arms and pull the weights up to your shoulders and then slowly lower them back to your thighs. For variation, alternate your arms or perform the exercise with your palms facing inwards.

Waist: side bends

Stand with your feet apart, arms relaxed and pelvis tilted up. Allow your arms to hang straight down at your sides, hands grasping the weights, palms facing your thighs. Slowly bend from your waist to the left side, lifting your right hand to underarm while bending your right elbow. Then slowly repeat to the other side. Avoid bending over or arching your back.

Walking back to fitness

Even if you can't get to a gym, walking is one of the most effective ways of getting back into shape. It has also become one of the most popular activities at spas these days because it is so easy to take home and to fit it into your everyday life. From a gentle hike to a brisk paced walk, you can choose the style that suits your needs and vary it as you desire. At the Golden Door, California, USA, the morning hike is one of the most exhilarating ways you could wish to start the day. After a week of morning hikes and brisk walks at The Door, I came home feeling fit enough to enter the next Olympics, well almost. And even if you don't live in such beautiful surroundings, you can find a local park or head for the countryside at the weekend to get your walking fix.

The most natural form of exercise, done on a regular basis, walking can lower the risk of cardiovascular disease and osteoporosis, reduce body fat, tone muscle and increase overall stamina. Not only that, but because it is low impact, risk of injury is also low. You also need little in the way of equipment so you can exercise wherever you go.

The spa walking programme

WARM-UP
Always warm up with a 3-minute slow walk followed by some light stretching if needed. Drink water before, during and after walking.

GUIDELINES
• Avoid a bouncy, bobbing motion when you walk.
• When walking uphill, take smaller steps and maintain good alignment.
• Take smaller steps when walking downhill. Soften knees to decrease impact.
• Progress gradually.

WALKING TECHNIQUES

Basic walking (strolling up to 3.5 mph)
• Head in neutral position with chin parallel to ground, eyes looking ahead.
• Shoulders down, back, and relaxed, chest lifted.
• Keep pelvis in neutral position while lengthening torso. Hands and arms are relaxed and moving in opposition to the legs in a long pendulum swing close to the body. Avoid crossing the midline of the body.
• Land on the heel and roll through the ball of the foot.
• Stride length is determined by your leg length, muscle tightness and degree of pelvic rotation.

Fitness walking (3.6 to 5 mph)
• Maintain good posture as in Basic Walking, but with a slight forward lean from the ankles.
• Keep elbows bent at about 90°. Avoid crossing the midline of the body with the hands and do not swing the hands higher than top of chest. On the back swing, bring elbows slightly behind the body, hand to front of hip. Keep hands relaxed.
• Movement of the arms is produced at the shoulders, not the elbows. Keep elbows close to the body.
• Speed up arm swing to increase walking speed.
• Hips rotate slightly – this is a natural motion.
• Land mid-heel with the forefoot raised. Roll from heel to the ball of the foot. The knees are almost fully extended but do not lock.

Modified race walking (5 mph plus)
• Maintain the same posture as Fitness Walking. Increase speed of arms and legs.
• Hands should not reach further back than the buttocks on the back swing.
• Walk with feet closer together. This results in a natural hip rotation.
• Keep ball of rear foot on ground until the heel of forward leg has contacted the ground.
• Avoid hyper-extending the knee joint.

COOL DOWN

Always cool down for 3 to 5 minutes, then perform some of the static stretches below.

STATIC STRETCHES

Waist and upper back

With one hand on your hip, reach the other arm over your head while bending to the opposite side from the waist. Keep hips still. Hold for 10 to 30 seconds. Perform 1 to 2 times on each side.

Chest and front shoulder

Stand with your feet a shoulder-width apart. Clasp your hands behind your back with palms inwards. Press your hands towards the floor, bringing your shoulders down and back (a). Hold for 10 to 30 seconds. Perform 1 to 2 times.

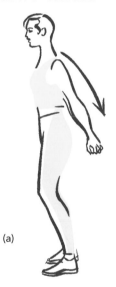

(a)

Hip and back

Stand tall. Place one hand under your left thigh and bring the top of the thigh towards your chest. Place the other hand against a wall for support. Circle the raised ankle 5 times inwards, then 5 times outwards. Switch sides.

Front thigh (quadriceps)

With your right hand holding your right ankle, bend your right knee and bring your heel towards your buttocks, keeping your opposite hand on a wall for stability if necessary. Keep your knees close together, hips pressed forwards and body upright. Repeat on the other side. Hold for 10 to 30 seconds. Perform 1 to 2 times on each leg.

Rear thigh (hamstring)

Stand with one heel on the ground or elevated on a step with the leg straight and the other leg 30 to 60 cm away from the step, knee bent. Press your hips backwards while keeping your back straight (b). Hold for 10 to 30 seconds. Perform 1 to 2 times on each leg.

Calf (calf stretch)   (b)

Step forwards, bend your front knee and press back the heel to the floor. Keep your back leg straight and toe pointing forwards. Then bring your rear foot slightly closer to your front foot and bend the back knee while keeping your heels down and body weight over the rear foot. Hold for 10 to 30 seconds each position. Perform 1 time on each leg.

WHAT TO LOOK FOR IN A WALKING SHOE

1 Low cut.
2 Bevelled heel.
3 Achilles notch
4 Flexible forefoot.
5 Light weight.
6 Roomy toe box.
7 Good heel stability.
8 Adequate cushioning.

THE SPA face
AND body blitz

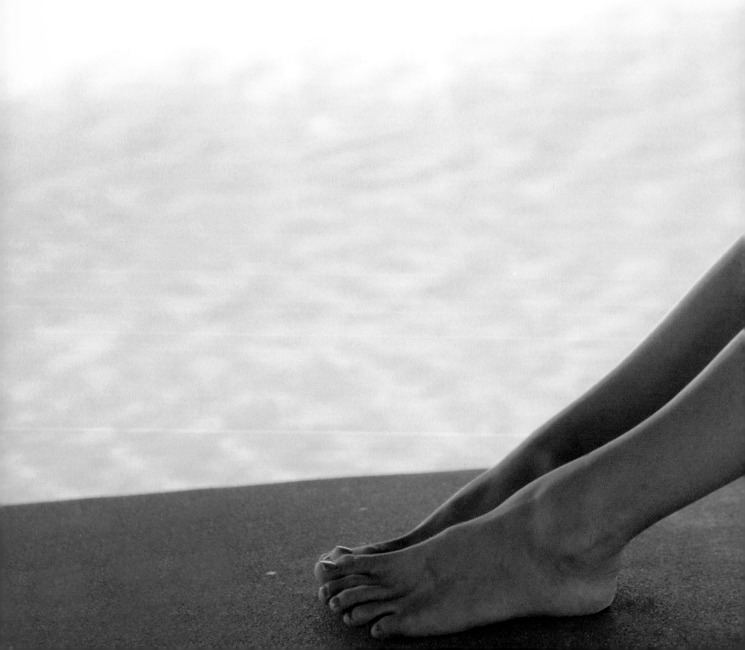

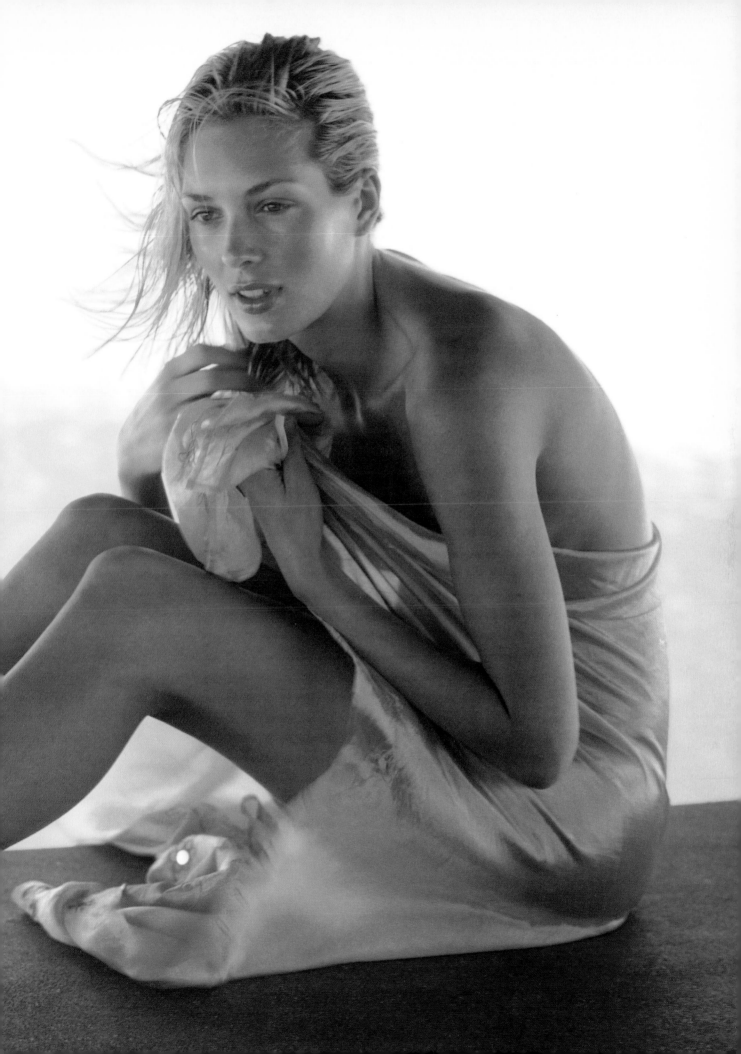

Body buffing

Exfoliating, sloughing, polishing – call it what you will. Although our skin naturally renews itself every 28 or so days and sheds any dead skin cells naturally, it always benefits from a helping hand. One of the most invigorating and instantly gratifying spa and salon treatments, body buffing not only leaves skin smooth-as-a-baby, but helps to rev up circulation and stimulate the lymphatic system – the body's natural waste disposal unit. While it's a blissful treat to have this done for you, it is equally rewarding at home. We've gathered some of the best body polishing recipes and techniques from spas around the globe.

Native body glow

Boost circulation with this remineralising and refreshing scrub from Vista Clara Ranch Resort and Spa, New Mexico, USA, that uses traditional Native American ingredients.

1 cup Dead Sea salts (available from health food shops and pharmacies)
50 g wholemeal flour
125 ml carrier oil such as almond oil
5 drops sage or cedarwood essential oil

1 Mix the ingredients in a small bowl set beside your bathtub. Shower to dampen skin and apply the mixture to your entire body, one section at a time.
2 Massage gently on freshly shaved areas and more vigorously on rough places, such as elbows, knees and feet. Don't leave on your skin for more than 5 minutes.
3 Rinse thoroughly. The result? Super-smooth, soft skin. Do not repeat more than two times weekly.

Salt body scrub

Pep up circulation and buff skin with this invigorating body polish from Lake Austin Resort, Texas, USA.

30 drops essential oils of lavender or rosemary
125 ml vegetable oil
50 g Dead Sea salts

1 Mix the essential oils with the vegetable oil and then add the Dead Sea salts. Blend thoroughly. Choose lavender oil for a relaxing blend or rosemary oil for a refreshing mix.
2 Use the mixture to scrub and exfoliate the body, ensuring that your skin is pre-showered and still damp, working upwards from the ankles. Rinse and pat skin dry gently. The result? Tingling refreshed skin.

Coconut body glow

This gentle body scrub from The Mandara Spa at The Chedi, Bali, Indonesia, is the perfect scrub for delicate skins as it exfoliates effectively but without causing irritation.

½ coconut, grated
¼ tsp turmeric powder or freshly grated turmeric root
250 g carrots, grated
2 tbsp gelatin powder

1 Mix the freshly grated coconut with the turmeric and gently rub over damp skin. Leave on for 5 minutes, then wipe off with a warm cloth.
2 Mix the carrot and gelatin together and apply to the skin. Leave for a few minutes then rinse off. The result? Skin feels smoother and moister.

Body polish

This exotic body scrub, created by spa beauty company Li'Tya for Daintree Eco-Lodge and Spa, Queensland, Australia, combines indigenous ingredients.

4 tbsp natural yoghurt
12 macadamia nuts, finely ground
2 tbsp elder flowers, ground (available from herbalists)
4 eucalyptus leaves, finely chopped (or 8 drops eucalyptus essential oil)

1 Combine the natural yoghurt, finely ground Macadamia nuts, ground elder flowers and finely chopped eucalyptus leaves or essential oils.
2 Rub into your body, massaging well to ensure full absorption. Wipe your skin clean with a warm, damp cloth.

Oriental body glow

Stimulate your circulation and soften your skin with this traditional Thai body scrub recipe from the Banyan Tree Spa, Phuket, Thailand.

250 ml runny honey
50 g sesame seeds
1 tsp dried herbs, such as mint or lavender leaf

1 Blend together the ingredients to make a thick paste.
2 Massage it into your skin from top to toe, working slowly and steadily so that your skin tingles. Finish by showering with warm water. The result? Gorgeously caramel-scented skin that is satiny-smooth.

Bali kopi scrub

For one of the most unusual sensory experiences, try this skin-smoothing, mouth-watering exfoliant, found at many of the premiere Far Eastern spas, such as The Mandara Spas at The Datai, Malaysia, and The Chedi, The Ibah, Bali Padma and Nikko, Bali, Indonesia.

200 g coffee beans, ground
3 tbsp kaolin clay (available at health food stores and pharmacies)
¼ tsp of ground pumice stone (optional)
250 g carrots, grated
1 tsp gelatin, already set (optional)
water

1 Grind the coffee beans finely and mix with the kaolin clay and ground pumice, if using. Add enough water to make a paste.
2 Rub over damp skin, allow to dry for a few minutes, then rub off vigorously.
3 Follow by rubbing in the carrot mixed with the gelatin (if using), which acts as a moisture replenisher. Shower and pat skin dry. The result? Amazingly silky skin, deliciously scented with the aroma of coffee.

Soothing baths

Now part and parcel of most spa beauty programmes, aromatherapy has been used by many ancient cultures as part of a well-being ritual. In aromatherapy, essential oils extracted from flowers and plants are used in massage, inhalation and bathing to benefit mind, body and spirit. When using them in the bath, stick to the recommended dose as they are very potent.

Herbal baths and treatments have become more popular at conventional spas and can now be found on most menus. For home treatments, herbs can be purchased from a wide number of herbalist suppliers (see stockists). As with essential oils, do seek medical advice before using them, especially orally.

You can use herbs to make tisanes and infusions to drink and for the bath. When you are using them in the bath, put the loose herbs in a muslin bag (available from most herbal suppliers) or simply place a handful in the middle of a muslin cloth square and tie up like a knapsack to prevent herbs escaping. Place the bag under the hot tap as you run the bath or leave to steep for a few minutes before you get in.

GUIDELINES
• If you do suffer from any serious medical condition or are pregnant, consult your doctor or midwife before using essential oils.
• Although there are a huge number of oils available on the high street and in supermarkets, cheap may be cheerful but in the case of essential oils, sadly, you pay for quality (see stockists for suggested reputable suppliers).

Desert journey tea bath

Evocative of the tranquillity and aromas of the south west, this luxurious bath treat from Westward Look Resort, Arizona, USA, is guaranteed to leave you feeling calm and at one with nature. The Desert Journey Bath Tea itself is available direct from the spa (see directory) or you can make a similar recipe as follows.

1 tbsp each of rose petals, citrus peel, lavender, rosemary, chamomile and sage
10 drops lavender essential oil

1 Add the lavender to the herbs and store in a glass jar, preferably dark glass. If you can't find a dark glass jar, store in a clear glass container away from the light.
2 Shake to mix thoroughly and add 2 heaped tablespoons to a muslin bag or cloth. Steep for a few minutes in a comfortably warm bath, light some candles and put on some soothing music. Westward Look's spa director, Lydia Corona, suggests listening to some Native American flute music – check out anything by R. Carlos Nakai (see page 23).

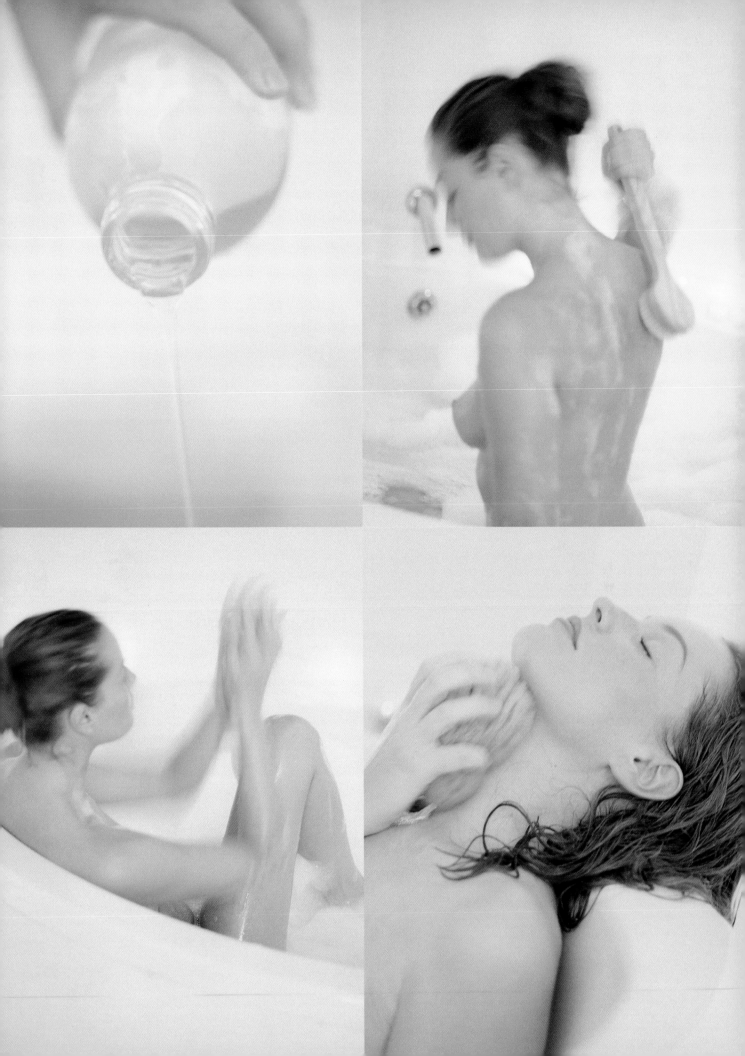

Restorative herbal bath

For a luxurious soak, try this herbal bath from The Spa at The Hyatt Regency-Coolum, Queensland, Australia.

herbal bag (see below for recipe)
Coral Moon bath oils (see below for recipes)
cold eucalyptus fragranced towel
rolled towel for head
measuring cup for oils

1 Fill your bath with warm water and, while the bath is running, add the bag of herbs. Choose your oil dependent on your mood (see below) and add to the bath. Light some candles, turn on your most relaxing music and settle into the bath. Steep for 30 minutes with a nice glass of wine.

RESTORATIVE HERBAL BAG
2 tablespoons each of lemon balm, lemon verbena, citronella grass, marigold flowers, geranium flowers, mint leaves and 50 g of oats. Place in a glass jar to store. Add a handful to a muslin bag or cloth and steep in warm bath water.

CORAL MOON OILS
Tension and stress relieving: 4 drops each of geranium, clary sage, rose, frankincense
Relaxing: 4 drops each of chamomile, lavender, orange, petitgrain
Refreshing: 4 drops each of peppermint, lemon, bergamot.

Cleansing bath

To detoxify mind and body, try this cleansing bath, inspired by the detoxifying aromatherapy baths offered at many Asian spas.

ginger, sage and rosemary essential oils
1 tbsp almond or jojoba oil

1 Add 3 drops each of the essential oils to a warm bath, just before you step into the bath. Inhale deeply, lie back and soak for 20 minutes.
2 Dry your skin thoroughly and then massage the same combination of oils blended with the almond or jojoba oil into your skin. Wrap up in a warm towelling robe and climb into bed. Rest for at least half an hour.
3 To complete the process, drink 6-8 glasses of water throughout the day, or if you are going straight to bed, sip a cup of fennel herbal tea.

Hot aroma bath soak

For a soothing bath, try this recipe from the Golden Door, California, USA, created by Cindy Fitzgerald from the spa's beauty department.

Choose your favourite flower, be it roses, gardenias or lavender, and put two cupfuls of dried flowers into a cheesecloth and allow to steep for a few minutes in a hot tub. Once infused, step in and soak for at least 20 minutes.

Thalassotherapy treat

The basis of many curative programmes at European and Japanese spas, thalassotherapy uses the healing power of water. In thalassotherapy (from the Greek thalassa, meaning sea), sea water and marine extracts are used in a variety of treatments from underwater massage to body wraps. The first modern thalassotherapy centre was set up by Dr Rene Bagot at Roscoff in Brittany, and since then, centres have been set up along the French coast at locations such as Deauville and Quiberon and on the African Atlantic at Casablanca. Bagot discovered that the minerals and trace elements present in sea water were almost identical to those found in our own blood plasma. By heating up the sea water, our bodies can absorb these minerals by osmosis.

Inspired by the sea water and seaweed enriched baths at the Hotel Miramar's Institute of Thalassotherapy Louison Bobet, Biarritz, France, this restorative soak will boost flagging energy levels and help to detoxify.

100 g dried or micronised seaweed
125 ml very hot water
3 drops lavender essential oil

1 Dissolve the dried or micronised seaweed (available from health food stores, spas and beauty salons) in the very hot water and add to a bath heated to 38°C.
2 Add the lavender essential oil just before you step in and soak for at least 20 minutes. Wrap up warmly after you dry yourself and try to drink as much water as possible to aid the elimination process.

Therapeutic bath

For a restorative spa bath, similar to those found at the spa at Baden in Austria, ensure that water is between 36 and 38°C to aid relaxation. Shower first with warm water, then run a warm bath. To soothe frazzled nerves, add a handful of valerian; to ease tension, try chamomile and to stimulate sluggish circulation, add rosemary. Place the herbs in a muslin or cheesecloth and tie with string. Dunk in the water and allow to steep for at least 5 minutes before you get in. While your bath is running, take a handful of damp sea salt (see Body Buffing recipes) blended with a little oil and massage into your skin. Slip into the bath and soak for at least 20 minutes.

Refreshing sitz bath

One of the staples at Austrian, German and Hungarian spas, sitz baths help to promote restful sleep, encourage relaxation and stimulate circulation and digestion. Fill your bath with enough warm water to allow you to sit in the tub with the water level with your waist. Add 6 to 8 drops of a refreshing essential oil such as mandarin, tangerine, lemon balm or peppermint, wrap your torso in a warm towel and soak for about 10 minutes. Finish with a cool top-to-toe shower.

Power shower

If you have a high-pressure shower at home, try this invigorating hydrotherapy treatment based on a treatment at the Blitzguss spa. Take a warm shower first, then switch to cold water and spray areas prone to poor circulation and cellulite, such as thighs, bottom, hips and upper arms, for 20 seconds at a time, before switching back to warm for 1 or 2 minutes, then back to cold water for a final spritz. Work your way up the body, starting with your legs. For a general tonic and immune-system boost, use the same technique to spray your whole body, starting with your face, then moving on to arms, chest, stomach, back, bottom, legs and feet. Finish with a brisk rub with a sisal mitt and pat skin dry with a fluffy towel.

Body wraps and packs

Body wraps, mud packs and masks come in a variety of guises. From the exotic experience of a rose oil body or papaya wrap to the deep-cleansing benefits of a seaweed, kaolin or Fuller's earth pack, there's a recipe for every skin requirement. You can adapt the recipes to suit your own personal preferences and needs, adding a little honey for extra moisture or specific essential oils to treat problem zones. With endless possibilities, you'll never get bored. To get you started, try these restorative wraps and packs, available at some of the world's foremost spas.

Aromatic body pack

This deep cleansing earth pack is similar to body packs available at many Middle Eastern and Asian spas. Particularly recommended for problem skins and those suffering from blemished backs, the clay or Fuller's earth helps to absorb impurities and encourage healing.

150 g green clay or Fuller's earth (available from health food stores and pharmacies)
220 ml water
2 tbsp organic clear honey
2 drops frankincense essential oil
2 drops vetiver essential oil
4 drops lavender or rose essential oil

1 Mix the clay or Fuller's earth with the water and blend into a smooth paste.
2 Add the honey and essential oils and apply to required areas. Leave on for 15 minutes, then shower off with warm water. Pat the skin dry.

Essential rose body wrap

Indulge in this nourishing and deliciously scented body treatment originating from the Lake Austin Spa Resort, Texas, USA. At the spa, skin is exfoliated with ground olive stones, then smothered in organic essential oil of rose and wrapped in layers of thermal blankets. Finally, frankincense and rose essential oils are massaged into the skin for gentle stimulation of blood flow and lymphatic circulation. The result? Removal of dead cells and dry skin, improvement in skin tone and texture, and a feeling of being rested, calmed and deeply relaxed.

body scrub (see pages 86-7 for recipes)
125 ml carrier oil, such as almond, avocado or jojoba oil
rose essential oil
plastic sheet
warm blankets
hot-water bottle
frankincense essential oil

1 Exfoliate your skin with a body scrub and shower off with warm water. Pat skin dry.
2 Add the rose oil to 125 ml of carrier oil and smooth on to your skin from top to toe. Save the leftover oil for the next step of the treatment. Wrap up in a plastic sheet and blankets and have a hot-water bottle at your feet. Relax for 15 to 20 minutes.
3 Add the frankincense oil to the leftover rose and carrier oil blend. Finish by massaging your body with the oil and leave it to soak in before dressing.

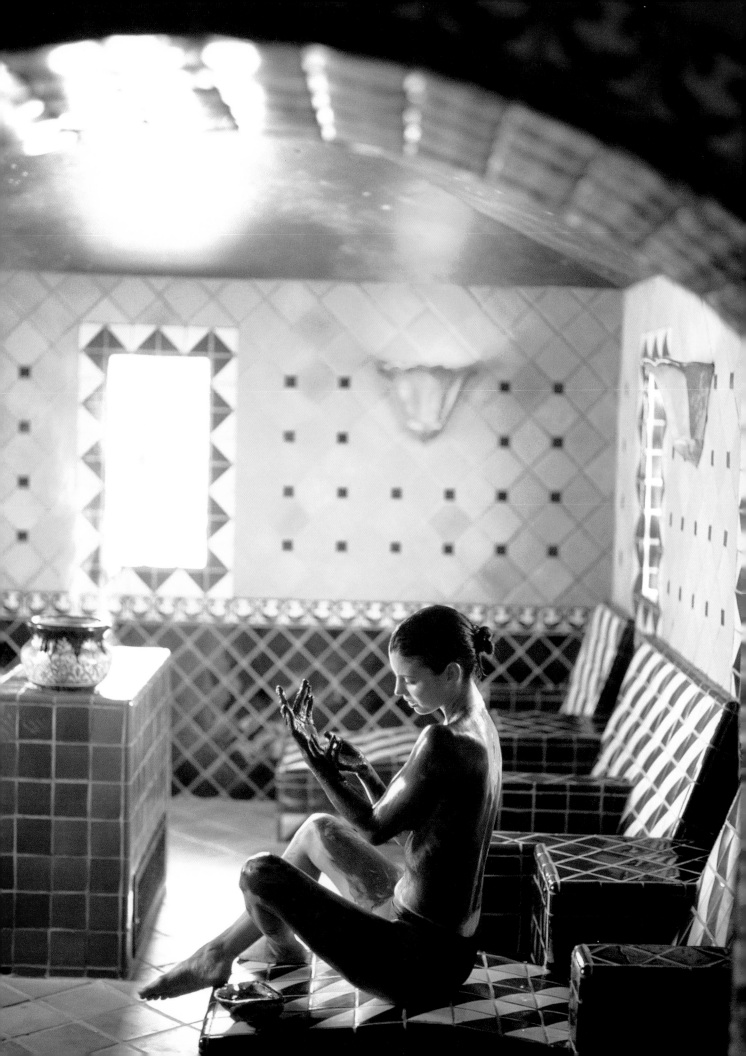

Aloe and lavender wrap

This has to be one of the most skin-soothing treatments available East or West. Adapted from a recipe from The Jimbaran Spa at The Four Seasons Resort, Bali, Indonesia, this will take your skin from dehydrated to deliciously moisturised. At the Jimbaran, the treatment also involves using banana leaves but as these are not too easy to come by, use a cotton sarong or sheet instead.

1 tsp fresh aloe pulp (plants are available from most garden centres and florists)
10 tbsp aloe vera gel (available from health food stores)
lavender essential oil
125 ml distilled water
juice of 4 lemons or limes
450 ml warm water
body lotion

1 Mix the fresh aloe with the aloe vera gel and apply to your body.
2 Add 10 drops of the lavender oil to the distilled water and pour into an atomiser and spray over your body.
3 Lie down and place a cotton sarong gently over you. Relax for about 20 minutes.
4 Add the lemon or lime juice to the 450 ml of warm water. Also add 4 drops of the lavender essential oil. Shower with warm water, then splash your body with the lime or lemon juice water.
5 Rinse again with warm water, pat skin dry, then massage in a generous amount of your favourite body lotion.

Papaya body mask

A legendary body treat at Far Eastern spas, including The Oriental Spa, Bangkok, Thailand, papaya contains papain, an enzyme that helps to soften skin and aid digestion. It is also a natural source of AHAs (alpha hydroxy acids), which help to exfoliate the skin.

2 ripe papayas
2 drops mandarin essential oil
2 drops vetiver

1 Blend the ripe papayas in a food processor until smooth, then add the mandarin essential oil and vetiver.
2 Apply to your body and wrap up in a plastic sheet for 20 minutes. Rinse off with warm water.

Body mud

This purifying body mask is a favourite at Daintree Eco-Lodge and Spa, Queensland, Australia.

1 tsp dried seaweed
250 ml water
2 tbsp kaolin clay
1 tbsp rose water
2 tbsp macadamia oil
1 tbsp clear organic honey
1 drop peppermint essential oil
2 drops sandalwood essential oil
1 drop lavender essential oil
1 drop sage essential oil

1 Boil the dried seaweed in the water for 5 minutes and then leave to cool.
2 Combine the kaolin, rose water and macadamia oil with the honey. Add the peppermint, sandalwood, lavender and sage essential oils and combine thoroughly
3 Smooth over your body. Keep the body wrapped or warm for 10 to 15 minutes and then rinse off with warm water.

Detox

If the word detox sends shivers down your spine, listen up. When it comes to an instant body overhaul, a detox cannot only be satisfying but a pleasurable ritual. Created by the experts at The Spa at St David's Hotel, Cardiff, UK, try the detox routine given below, guaranteed to sweep away any cobwebs, uplift your spirits, boost your energy levels and leave you feeling ultra-clean.

DETOX ROUTINE

Step 1: brush skin
Using light, upward movements, stroke your skin with a sisal body brush or hemp mitt, always working towards the heart. Stroke each part of the body three times, working from the soles of your feet upwards. Body brushing helps to stimulate the body's lymphatic system, helping to reduce fluid retention and, some experts believe, cellulite.

Step 2: shower
Put 3 to 4 drops of peppermint essential oil on to a sisal pad or hemp mitt. Massage this into your skin as you shower in comfortably warm water. Work upwards from the ankles, using small, brisk, circular movements.

Step 3: exfoliate
Use a handful of sea salt mixed with a tablespoon of body oil to buff damp skin. Use circular movements, again working from the feet, upwards. Pat the skin dry and wrap up warmly in a towelling robe or loose clothing.

Daintree body brush

For an invigorating, detoxifying experience, try this body brushing routine from Daintree Eco-Lodge and Spa, Queensland, Australia. Not only will it help to remove dead skin cells but also it stimulates blood circulation. Ideally, body brushing should be done every morning before showering or bathing.
• Using the body brush on your legs, make upward stokes towards the heart following with your free hand.
• Use the same method on the arms.
• Stroke the back, three movements on the right side, then the middle and then strokes on the left side of the back. (You may need assistance!)
• Use fast upward movements on the buttocks to get the blood flowing (it's great for cellulite).
• Use circular, clockwise strokes on the stomach.
• Then shower or soak in a warm bath. Moisturise the body with your favourite lotion or oil.

Deep cleansing body rub

Cleanse and detoxify skin with this stimulating rub, inspired by traditional Far Eastern spa recipes.

2 tbsp ground sandalwood powder
4 tbsp goat's milk yoghurt
2 tsp honey

1 Mix the ground sandalwood powder with the goat's milk yoghurt and honey and massage vigorously into damp skin.
2 Leave on for 15 to 20 minutes, then rinse off with warm water. The result is glowing, fresh-looking skin.

Deluxe body treats

There are some spa body recipes that deserve to be dubbed deluxe. Here are a few of my own favourite indulgences, from the sublime Petals body treatment at Ojai Valley Inn and Spa, California, which makes you feel like you're in heaven, to the delectable vinotherapie from the Caudalie Institut in France. Prepare to experience Nirvana …

Petals

The signature body treatment at the Ojai Spa, California, USA, is one of life's most delicious pampering experiences. Based on soothing, nurturing essential rose oils known for its calming, romantic and healing effects, Petals comprises three parts: exfoliation, showering and moisturising. At the Ojai Spa, Jurlique products are used, but you can substitute any good quality rose oils.

25 g corn starch
25 g corn meal
20 drops rose geranium essential oil
12 drops rose absolute essential oil
shower gel
rose essential oil
body lotion or massage oil

1 Begin by exfoliating the skin with a mixture of the corn starch, corn meal, rose geranium essential oil and rose absolute essential oil. Combine all the ingredients and place in a shaker jar (like a sugar shaker with wide holes in the lid).
2 Sprinkle on the skin and gently exfoliate to remove the dead cells from the surface of the skin.
3 Shower in warm but not too hot water with a shower gel to which you have added 10 drops of rose essential oil.
4 Finally, smooth on a lotion or massage oil containing rose essential oil. Let the oil remain on the skin for at least a few hours. The effect is amazing: your skin will feel satiny soft and you will smell divine.

Vinotherapie body treat

At the Caudalie Institut de Vinotherapie, Martillac, France, treatments are based on grapes and wine. Both are rich sources of anti-oxidant polyphenols. Try this 'at home' body treatment using the Caudalie Vinotherapie philosophy. Blend 20 fresh grapes with 5 teaspoons of organic honey and 10 teaspoons of body scrub (see Body Buffing section for a selection of recipes) to make a paste. Massage it into damp skin and shower off. Pat your skin dry and finish by massaging your body from top to toe with grape-seed oil to which you have added vetiver or petitgrain essential oil.

Agua milk and honey

This is my all-time favourite indulgence, based on an ancient ayurvedic recipe by spa creators Rita Shrager and Leila Fazel, responsible for Agua at Delano, Florida, USA, and more recently, Agua at Sanderson, London, UK.

4 tbsp powdered milk
3 tbsp organic clear honey
1 tbsp sesame oil

1 Combine the milk powder with enough hot water to create a thin, smooth paste.
2 Combine the honey and sesame oil and heat gently in a bain-marie or microwave until warm.
3 Apply the honey and oil mixture to as much of your body as possible using a sweeping massage movement. Lie down on a towel or cotton sheet and leave on for 10 minutes.
4 Remove the honey and oil mixture with the warm milk paste and a washcloth. The milk not only helps the sticky honey to glide off, but is excellent nourishment for the skin.

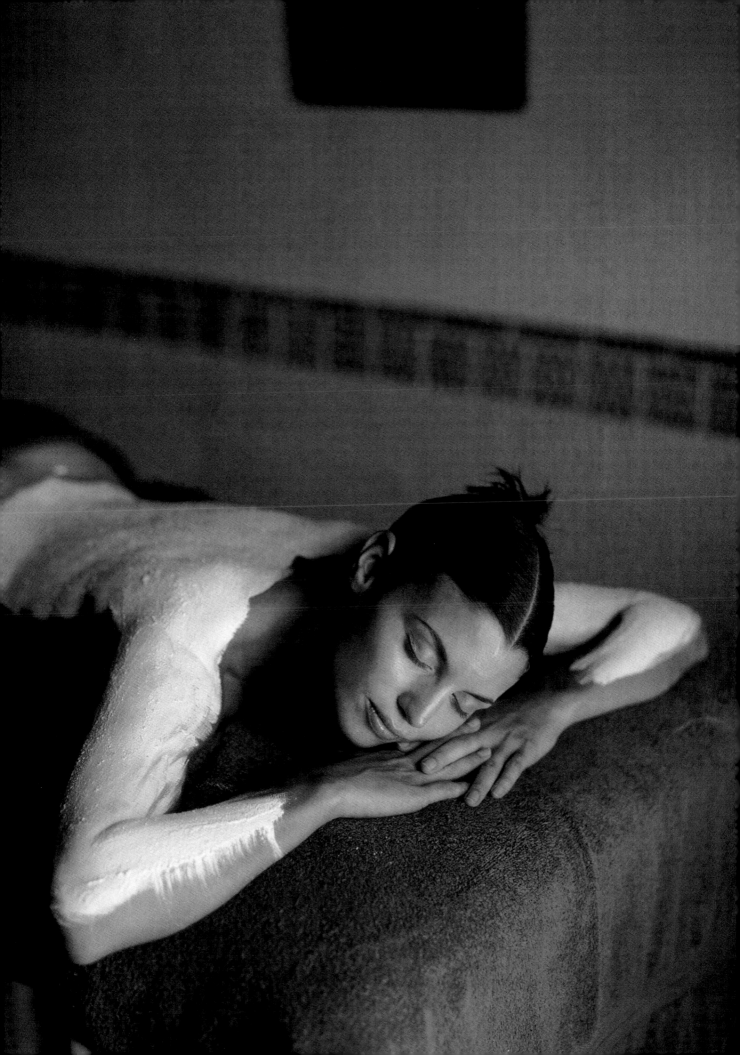

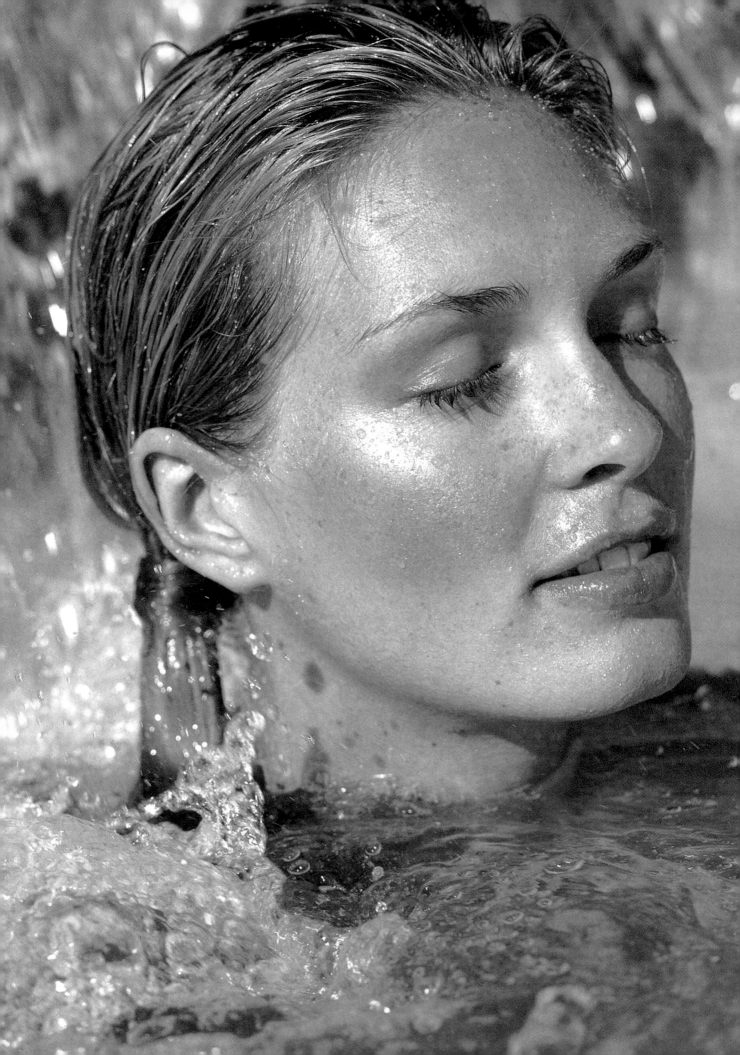

Spa treats for your face

While the focus of most spas is inner rather than outer beauty, no matter where they happen to be located across the globe, the majority of modern spas offer a mind-boggling array of facial pampering. Masks, scrubs, massage and skin boosters, spa menus boast a host of beautifying treatments designed to restore our city-weary complexions to their former glory.

While there is no doubt that having a facial is one of the most wonderfully soothing therapies, you can reap some of the benefits of spa beauty wisdom at home. From traditional Malaysian and Balinese preparations to replenishing masks and scrubs from as far afield as Australia and Arizona, skin maintenance need never be mundane again. And if, like me, you are pushed for time, there are fast-track treats from a 5-minute face mask to a 10-minute Shiatsu massage so that even when time is tight, you can still look groomed and feel pampered.

FACIAL MASSAGE

Nothing boosts circulation better than a facial massage. The basis of many spa facials, massage is key when it comes to maintaining skin tone as we age. For a once-a-week treat, use the following routine on freshly cleansed skin. Always use an oil when you massage to avoid dragging your skin and to allow your fingertips to move easily over your face and neck.

1 Choose your massage oil to suit your current skin type. You can add three to four different essential oils to your chosen carrier oil. Start by warming a teaspoon of oil in your palms, rub your hands together briskly, then press them over your face, starting at your forehead and working your way outwards and upwards with firm pressure.
2 Next, use your fingertips to lightly tap all around your face. Start by tapping around your brows, underneath your eyes, along your cheekbones, under your nose and around your mouth and along your jaw, always starting from the centre of your face and working outwards.
3 Add a little more oil to your palms, rub your palms together and use your fingertips to massage your face with small circular movements, again starting at your brows, working around your eye sockets, across the cheekbones to your ears and so on.
4 Add more oil and work from the base of your neck upwards to your chin and jaw line, using your fingers in sweeping movements.
5 Finish by pressing your palms and heels of your hands across your face, as in step 1.

FACIAL OILS

The following oils can be used to dilute essential oils for facial massage. Use 30 ml of carrier oil to 10 drops of essential oil.

Apricot kernel oil: perfect for use on the face as it is light in texture and easily absorbed. Skin type: suits all skin types, but particularly good for dry skin.
Avocado oil: rich in vitamins A and B. Skin type: suitable for dry and sensitive skins.
Grape seed oil: rich in antioxidants, light in texture and easily absorbed. Skin type: suits oily to combination skins.
Jojoba oil: a very versatile, balancing oil. Skin type: can be used to treat psoriasis and eczema and works equally well on oily or acne-prone skins.
Sweet almond oil: one of the most widely used skin softeners. Skin type: great for all skin types.
Vitamin E oil: rich in anti-ageing antioxidants. Skin type: excellent for very dry, sun-damaged skins and skin that needs an intensive booster.

ESSENTIAL OILS

Always use a carrier or base oil when using essential oils, particularly on your face. Lavender and tea tree oil can be dabbed directly on to blemishes undiluted but those with sensitive skin should be very cautious.

Bergamot: antiseptic and astringent bergamot works to rebalance oily and blemished skin.

Chamomile: contains an ingredient called azulene that is known to be soothing and antibacterial.

Frankincense: excellent for very dry or mature skins, it is incredibly soothing.

Jasmine: suitable for most skin types, jasmine is a wonderful soother.

Lavender: can be dabbed on to blemishes as it has antibacterial and antiseptic properties.

Patchouli: effective moisturiser for very dry skin, is also antiseptic.

Rose: works for all skin types and has an antibacterial action.

Sandalwood: use to treat acne-prone skin and to rebalance very oily complexions.

Tea tree: excellent antiseptic and skin-healing properties. Like lavender, it can be dabbed on to blemishes neat.

AROMATIC FACIAL BLENDS

Try some of these evocative essential oil combinations.

Eastern serenity: blend 30 ml carrier oil, 3 drops patchouli essential oil, 2 drops sandalwood essential oil and 2 drops jasmine essential oil.

English rose: blend 30 ml carrier oil, 5 drops rose essential oil, 3 drops rose geranium oil, 2 drops lavender essential oil.

Tropical treat: blend 30 ml carrier oil, 4 drops mandarin oil, 2 drops neroli and 2 drops ylang ylang.

South-western breeze: blend 30 ml carrier oil, 4 drops sage oil, 2 drops cedarwood and 2 drops lavender.

SPECIAL RECIPES

Try these essential oil blends for treating specific skin conditions.

Skin hydrator for parched, dry skin: blend 30 ml of carrier oil with 3 drops of lavender oil, 2 drops of neroli oil and 2 drops of patchouli oil.

Instant purification for blemished skin: blend 30 ml of carrier oil with 3 drops of tea tree oil, 2 drops of chamomile oil, 2 drops of bergamot oil and 2 drops of lavender oil.

Wake-up treat for fatigued, lacklustre skin: blend 30 ml of carrier oil with 4 drops of sandalwood oil, 3 drops of jasmine oil and 3 drops of rose oil.

Post-sun reviver for over-exposed skin: blend 30 ml of carrier oil with 5 drops of chamomile and 5 drops of lavender.

Break-out blend for zapping blemishes: blend 15 ml of carrier oil with 5 drops of bergamot oil, 5 drops of tea tree oil and 5 drops of lavender oil. Dab on individual blemishes.

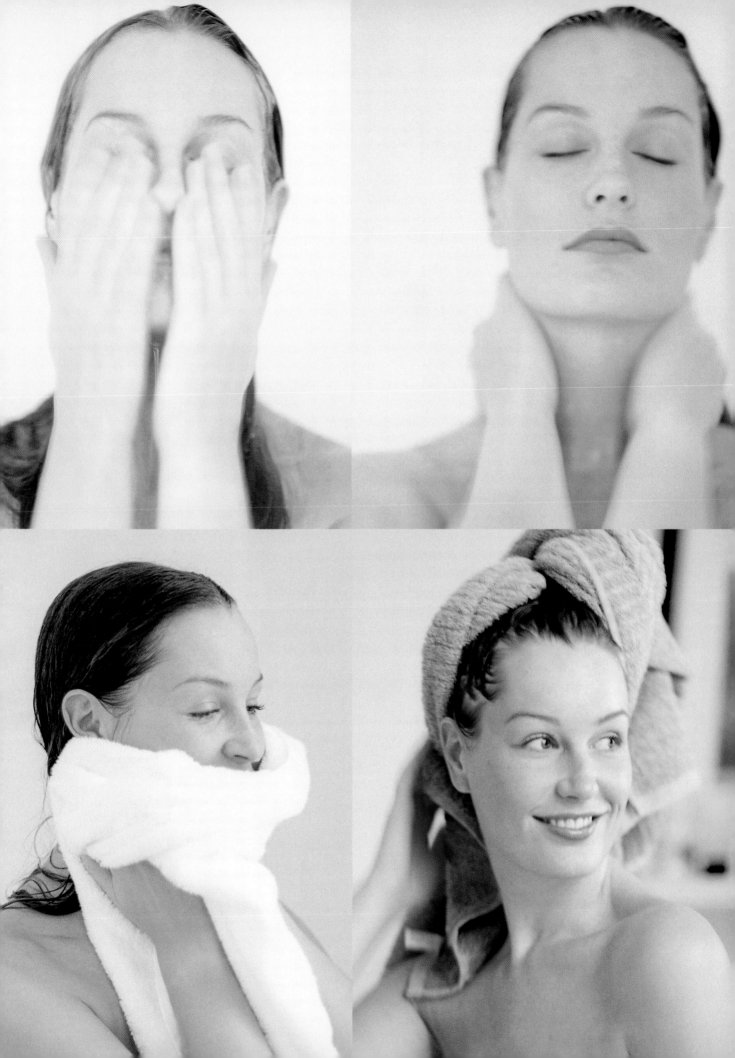

DIY facials

Even the dullest complexion will glow after this revitalising facial routine devised by spa company Li'Tya for Daintree Eco-Lodge and Spa, Queensland, Australia.

1 Cleanse

1 tsp juice of wild lime
1 tsp eucalyptus gum honey
1 tsp lemon myrtle tea infusion (prepare 250 ml of tea, to be used during steaming and exfoliation processes, tea leaves as well as the tea liquor)
2 tbsp natural yoghurt
1 tbsp baked yam
1 drop wild lavender essential oil
1 drop mandarin essential oil

Blend all the ingredients in listed order, adding the essential oils last. Add a little more lemon myrtle tea infusion if the mixture is too thick.

2 Steam

2 litres boiling water
3 leaves lemon myrtle
3 leaves eucalyptus
1 tbsp fresh peppermint leaves or 2 drops peppermint essential oil

Dilute the remaining lemon myrtle tea infusion with the boiling water in a large bowl. Then add the rest of the ingredients to the infusion. Cover your head and the bowl with a large towel to receive maximum benefit from steaming. Remain under the steam for at least 5 minutes.

3 Exfoliate

1 tsp finely grated wild lime rind
1 tbsp eucalyptus gum honey
1 tsp ground macadamia nuts

Remove the lemon myrtle, eucalyptus and fresh peppermint leaves from the steam bowl and chop them finely. If the lemon myrtle tea infusion was made with a tea bag, add the contents to the mixture also. Then add the fresh ingredients listed above.

Massage the mixture gently on to your face and throat, taking care around the eye area. To remove, wet a face flannel with warm water and wipe your face. Rinse your face with a cool splash of water to complete this step. Pat dry with a clean towel.

4 Mask

2 tbsp cream (full fat content)
1 tbsp eucalyptus gum honey
2 tsp dried lavender flowers
2 tsp fresh jasmine flowers
1 tsp grated mandarin rind (optional)

Make a mixture from the ingredients, first whipping together the cream and honey. Add the flowers and mandarin rind and mix well before applying to your face. Leave the mask on your face for 15 to 20 minutes. To remove, wet a face flannel with warm water and wipe off gently.

5 Hydrate

Complete with applying a small amount of macadamia oil (or a light vegetable or nut oil) and blot out with a tissue.

Eastern facial

Is your skin in need of an overhaul? Try this deluxe facial inspired by recipes from Indonesian spas including The Mandara Spas at The Chedi, Bali, Indonesia and The Datai, Malaysia.

1 tbsp dry corn kernel
1 tbsp ground rice powder
2 tbsp clay powder
1 tbsp cucumber juice for oily skin or 15 ml carrot juice for normal/dry skin

1 For the scrub mix the corn kernels with the rice powder and add either cucumber or carrot juice depending on your skin type to make a scrub. Massage into damp, freshly cleansed skin.
2 Remove the scrub with warm water and a muslin cloth, massaging gently as you go.
3 Mix the clay and the carrot or cucumber juice to make a mask and use a pastry brush to brush it on to your face, avoiding the eye area.
4 Leave on for 10 to 15 minutes and remove with warm water and a muslin cloth.
5 Pat your skin dry and use a little rose or sandalwood facial oil to moisturise your skin, using your fingertips to tap lightly across your face to stimulate your circulation.

Traditional Thai facial

Simple ingredients yield potent results in this traditional Thai-style facial based on a recipe used for many centuries by Thai women. Variations are available at many Indonesian and Thai spas, including The Banyan Tree Spa, Bintan, Indonesia and The Banyan Tree Spa, Phuket, Thailand. PS: if you thought cucumbers were the staple of teenage beauty treatments, think again.

225 g clear honey
10 drops fresh lime juice
1 medium-sized cucumber, thinly sliced, rind removed

1 Cleanse your face with warm water and a muslin cloth.
2 Mix the honey and lime juice together and pat on to your face, massaging it in for 10 to 15 minutes.
3 Remove the honey with warm water and a muslin cloth.
4 Lie down, and place the cucumber slices over your entire face, allowing them to overlap.
5 Leave for 10 minutes while you relax and practise some deep breathing.
6 Rinse your skin with cool water and pat dry.
7 Finish by applying a little soya oil to moisturise.

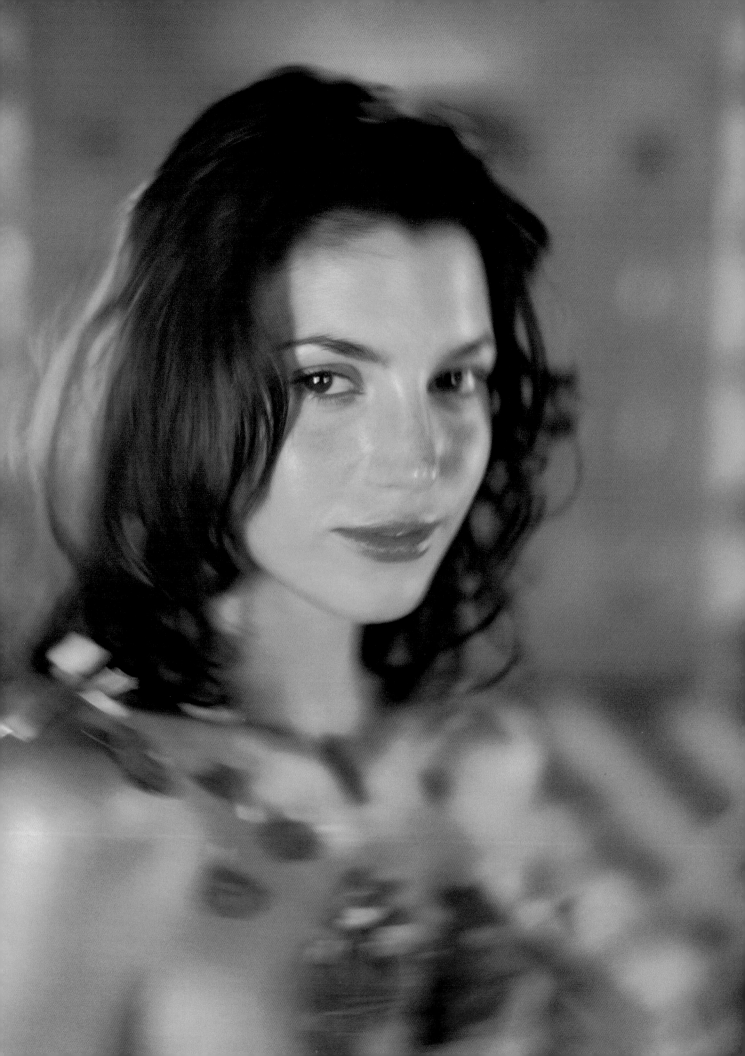

Cleansing and toning

Give your skin care routine a makeover with freshly made cleansers, masks and scrubs straight from the recipe books of spas across the globe. Not only do they prove that treating your skin can be fun rather than a chore, but that beauty doesn't have to cost the earth.

Yoghurt and polenta scrub

Gently slough away dead skin with this super-cleansing facial polish from The Mandara Spa at The Chedi, Bali, Indonesia.

2 tbsp natural yoghurt
1 tbsp polenta

1 Mix the yoghurt and polenta into a paste and gently rub into damp skin with your fingertips.
2 Work your way outwards, starting from the centre of your forehead to your hairline, down your nose and along your cheeks to your ears, and from your mouth and chin and across your jaw line.
3 Rinse away with warm water and a muslin cloth.

Tropical facial scrub

Treat skin to this tropical treat inspired by traditional Asian spa recipes and made with a combination of zingy citrus ingredients and delicious soothing honey and jasmine oil.

3 tbsp ground oatmeal or polenta
1 tsp freshly grated orange peel
1 tsp freshly squeezed lemon or lime juice
1 tsp clear honey
1 tsp coconut oil
2 drops jasmine oil

1 Combine all the ingredients in a blender until you have a smooth paste.
2 Massage into your skin using circular movements with your fingertips.
3 Rinse away with warm water.

Honey and oil cleanser

For a deep-cleansing experience, try this cleanser, inspired by a recipe from The Jamu Traditional Spa, Bali, Indonesia.

2 tsp clear honey
3 tsp olive or coconut oil
1 drop frankincense essential oil

1 Blend together the honey, oil and frankincense essential oil.
2 Apply to your face with your fingertips and massage in.
3 Leave on for 2 to 3 minutes, then rinse off with warm water.
4 Pat your skin dry.

Exotic neroli and patchouli cleanser

Synonymous with Bali, patchouli is renowned for its healing action on the skin, while neroli, a natural sedative, calms and soothes the skin.

25 ml sweet almond oil
25 ml jojoba oil
3 drops neroli essential oil
3 drops patchouli essential oil
25 g cocoa butter
15 g beeswax
25 ml orange flower water
0.6 ml borax (available from chemists)

1 Combine all the oils and cocoa butter in a bain-marie. Add the beeswax, a little at a time, and stir in until it melts.
2 Warm the orange flower water in a small milk pan and stir in the borax.
3 Add to the oil mixture and mix well. Leave to cool and thicken.
4 When cool, put into a dark glass jar. Keep in a fridge and use within four weeks.
5 To use, just massage the mixture into your skin to dissolve traces of make-up and grime. Tissue off and finish off with a spritz of Lemon Refresher (see opposite for recipe).

Leila's peachy mask

Leila Fazel, co-creator of Agua at Delano, Florida, USA, and Agua at Sanderson, London, UK, shares her all-time favourite facial treat based on a traditional recipe that she learned from her Iranian-born mother.

2 tbsp natural yoghurt
2 tbsp peeled and mashed peaches
½ tsp baking soda
1 drop hydrogen peroxide (optional)

1 Make a mixture of the yoghurt, peeled and mashed peaches, baking soda and hydrogen peroxide (if using). Apply the mixture to your face and let it dry while you sip some herbal tea.
2 Once dry, wipe away with a warm washcloth and moisturise with a very thin layer of soya oil.

Aloe and lavender cooler

Based on a facial recipe from The Jimbaran Spa at The Four Seasons Resort, Bali, Indonesia, this mask is ideal for weather-beaten skin.

60 ml aloe vera gel
5 drops lavender essential oil

1 Mix the aloe vera gel with the lavender oil.
2 Place in the fridge to chill for 20 minutes.
3 Apply to your face, avoiding the eye area and leave for 15 minutes.
4 Rinse off with tepid water.

Rosy tonic

This fragrant tonic is the perfect English-style toner for dry or mature skins.

150 ml distilled water
10 drops rose essential oil
5 drops glycerine
100 ml witch hazel

1 Combine all the ingredients in a dark glass bottle and shake well.
2 Transfer to an atomiser and store a little in the refrigerator for a refreshing spritz.

Aromatic honey toner

Reminiscent of traditional Malaysian skin tonics, this honey water leaves skin wonderfully refreshed.

¼ tsp clear honey
1 tsp cider vinegar
120 ml distilled water
2 drops neroli essential oil
1 drop ylang ylang essential oil
1 drop sandalwood essential oil

1 Add the honey, vinegar and 20 ml of the water to a bain-marie and heat gently until the honey has dissolved.
2 Pour into a dark glass bottle and add the essential oils and the remaining water.
3 Store in a cool place; it keeps for two weeks.
4 Splash on to your skin after applying a mask or scrub. Leave for 30 minutes before rinsing off.

Santa Fe-style spritzer

Based on the sage native to the area surrounding the Ten Thousand Waves' Japanese-style spa, New Mexico, USA, this toner will leave your skin feeling tingly and refreshed.

3 tbsp dried sage
3 tbsp ethyl alcohol
1.25 ml borax
2 tbsp witch hazel
10 drops glycerine
2 drops sage essential oil
2 drops juniper essential oil

1 Place the sage and the alcohol in a bowl, cover and leave for 10 to 14 days. Strain and save the liquid for the next stage.
2 Dissolve the borax in the witch hazel and stir in the sage liquid. Add the glycerine and essential oils and pour into a dark glass bottle. Keep in a cool place and shake before use.

Lemon refresher

Based on a traditional Balinese spa recipe, this citrus spritz is the ideal refresher for oily skins.

1 lemon or lime, juiced
2 tbsp distilled water

1 Strain the lemon or lime juice, add to the water and mix. Place in a plastic atomiser and chill in the refrigerator.
2 Spritz on to your skin after applying a mask or scrub.

Face your problems

Sometimes skin demands intensive care or special measures to bring it back into balance. Seasonal changes, hormonal swings, environmental factors and stress levels can all add up to out-of-control skin. Designed to combat everything from desert-dry skin to an overly oily complexion, here are some favourite spa skin-saving solutions.

Aromatic facial steam

Steam baths and saunas are synonymous with spas. Excellent for cleansing and decongesting, try this aromatic sauna, especially for skin that is unbalanced or is prone to blemishes.

2 drops tea tree essential oil
2 drops lavender essential oil
1 drop sage essential oil
1 sprig fresh rosemary

1 Cleanse your face and dab a little eye cream around your eyes to protect the skin and add some lip balm to your lips.
2 Fill a bowl with freshly boiled water and add the essential oils and fresh herbs.
3 Cover your head with a towel and place your face over the bowl, ensuring that you are not too close to the boiling water.
4 Steam for about 5 minutes.

Lip soother

If your lips feel as dry as the Mojave Desert, try this to-die-for lip balm recipe created by Cindy Fitzgerald at the Golden Door, California, USA.

3 tsp beeswax
3 tsp almond oil

1 In a small bain-marie, melt the beeswax.
2 Add the almond oil and mix well.
3 Pour into a small, thick glass jar and leave to cool.
4 Massage into your lips to rehydrate and soothe.

Instant calmer

Masks are part and parcel of many spa facials, not only because of their effective deep-cleansing action, but because they deliver ingredients to the skin quickly and effectively. Ideal for intensive care, this soothing mask is a boon if your skin is going through a period of unrest or is overly sensitive.

1 tsp green clay
1 tsp oatmeal
1 tsp ground almonds
3 tbsp orange flower water
½ tsp vitamin E oil
1 drop neroli essential oil
1 drop sandalwood essential oil

1 Blend the clay, oatmeal and almonds with the orange flower water to form a paste.
2 Add the vitamin E and essential oils and mix well.
3 Smooth on to your face, avoiding the eye area, and leave for 15 minutes.
4 Remove with warm water and a muslin cloth, pressing gently at first to loosen the mask.

Aromatic face saver

This recipe, created by Cindy 'Hilani' Woodward from the Golden Door, California, USA, calms, heals and comforts dry skin – the best of face savers.

60 ml aloe vera gel
1 vitamin E capsule
½ tsp vanilla extract or 2 drops vanilla essential oil

1 Pre-chill the aloe vera gel in the fridge.
2 Break open the vitamin E capsule and combine it with the vanilla extract or oil.
3 Whip all the ingredients together until frothy and apply to your face for 10 to 15 minutes.
4 Remove with warm water and a muslin cloth or flannel.

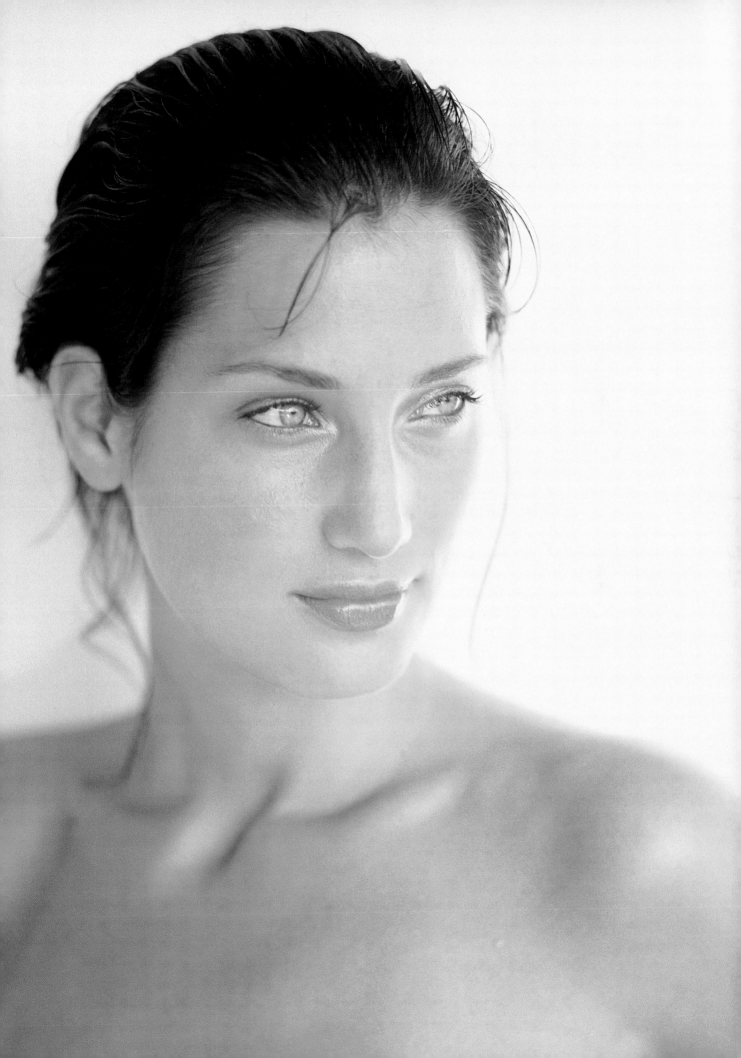

Hands and feet

Often neglected and always taken for granted, hands and feet are often the last to be indulged in pampering treats. Always included on spa menus, take your pick from these revitalising recipes and regimes.

Pampering pedicure

Created by Suzanne Chavez, spa therapy director at Vista Clara Ranch Resort and Spa, New Mexico, USA, this treatment will ensure the smoothest, sleekest feet.

1 basin or large bowl
1 litre warm to hot water
1 capful vinegar or 5 drops lavender essential oil

1 Find a comfortable chair and put on your favourite movie, radio programme or music.
2 Fill your pedicure tub with the warmest water you can tolerate.
3 Add the vinegar or lavender essential oil.
4 Soak your feet for at least 10 minutes.
5 Use your pedicure file to vigorously remove the rough edges on your feet. Place feet back in tub and soak again while you relax.
6 Then choose one of the ideas given below.

EXTEND YOUR PEDICURE

To relax: cover your feet entirely with a facial mask; prop up your feet wrapped in a warm, steamy, damp towel. When through, rinse and apply your favourite lotion.
To invigorate: combine enough salt and oil to mix easily and massage your feet thoroughly. Then dip your feet once again into the tub to rinse away the salt and pat dry.
To heal: apply comfrey salve or lavender oil and prop up your feet – relax – finish the movie!

Hand and wrist massage

Treat hands to this super-moisturising and relaxing massage, ideal for alleviating tension, particularly if you are working at a keyboard.

2 tsp sweet almond or jojoba oil
2 drops camomile essential oil
2 drops lavender oil

1 Blend all the ingredients together in a small cup. Place the cup in a bowl of boiling water, ensuring that the water level is about half-way down the cup. Let it stand for about 5 minutes to warm the oil.
2 Warm your hands by rubbing them briskly together or placing them in a bowl of warm water for a few minutes.
3 Pour the oil into your hands and massage it well into your wrists, palms and fingers, using firm, even pressure. Finish by patting your hands dry with a towel to remove excess oil.

Floral foot soak

Treat tired feet to this restorative footbath, based on the recipe from the spa at The Bali Hyatt, Bali, Indonesia.

125 ml of pre-blended foot scrub (see scrub recipe overleaf)
3 drops each of thyme, vetiver and sage essential oils
bowl of warm water
2 tbsp wheatgerm, coconut or jojoba essential oil
handful of fresh flowers

1 Scrub the feet with the foot scrub, rubbing vigorously to remove callused skin and to stimulate circulation. If you have very hard or rough skin, use a pumice stone with the scrub.
2 Rinse the feet under the shower. Pat dry.
3 Massage your feet with the **thyme, vetiver and sage essential oils**, working your way from the toes up to the ankles.
4 Fill a bowl with warm water and drop in the **wheatgerm, coconut or jojoba essential oil**. Throw in the flowers and place your feet in the bowl. Leave them to steep for 10 to 15 minutes.

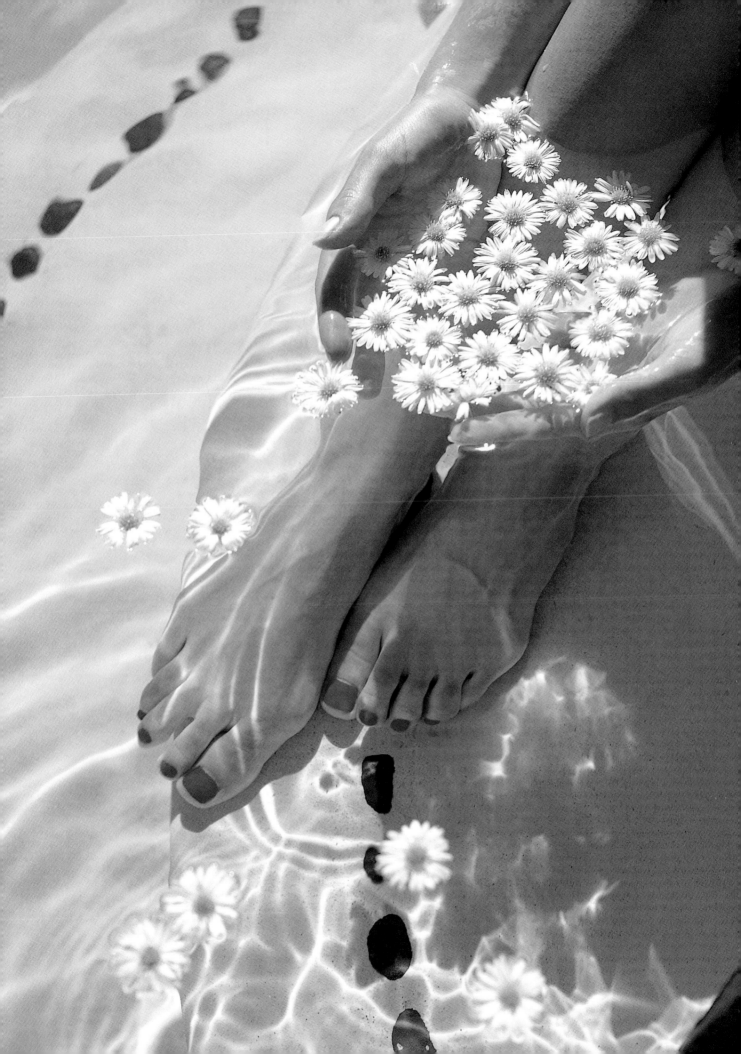

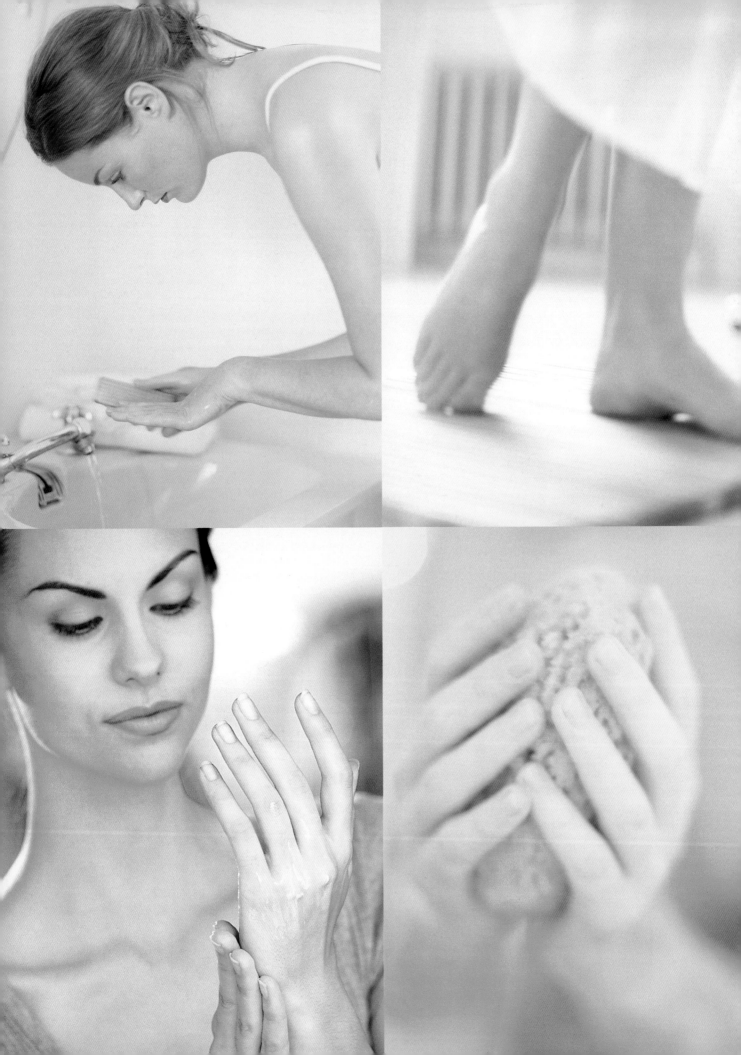

Flower mask for hands and feet

Based on a traditional Balinese spa recipe, this mask will deep cleanse and moisturise both hands and feet.

6 tbsp kaolin or green clay powder
2 tbsp coconut milk
1 tsp ground cloves
1 tsp ground cinnamon
1 tsp ground ginger
handful of rose petals or jasmine flowers
5 drops lavender essential oil

1 Combine all the ingredients to make a thick paste.
2 Apply to hands or feet and leave on for 20 minutes or until it dries.
3 Rinse with warm water, gently rubbing to remove traces of the mask.
4 Finish by massaging your hands or feet with coconut or sesame oil.

Nut scrub

Inspired by a recipe at The Jamu Traditional Spa, Bali, Indonesia, this foot scrub will leave feet feeling blissed out and super-smooth.

225 g lemon grass
500 ml boiling water
1 tbsp almonds
1 tbsp macadamia nuts
1 tsp coconut oil

1 Make an infusion with the lemon grass and boiling water. Let it steep for 20 minutes, cool, then strain and save the liquid in a jug.
2 Blend the nuts, lemon grass infusion and oil to make a smooth paste.
3 Massage into your feet to help remove dry skin.

Exotic hand cream

Try this super-moisturising recipe for parched hands which will leave skin soft and fragrant.

2 tsps honey
50 ml coconut oil
10 drops pure vitamin E oil
10 drops rose essential oil
10 drops sandalwood essential oil
5 drops ylang ylang essential oil

1 Warm the honey and coconut oil in a bain-marie and mix well until combined.
2 Add the vitamin E oil, then the essential oils.
3 Pour into a bowl and allow to cool to a comfortable temperature.
4 Massage into your hands and allow to soak in for at least 20 minutes before wiping away the excess with a warm, damp muslin cloth or towel.

All-over body boosters

Whether you are simply feeling under-the-weather or in need of a general boost, the following spa recipes are designed to zap specific problems, such as colds, aches and pains, fatigued muscles or skin that's playing up.

Immune booster bath

Inspired by treatments at Israeli spas, such as the Radisson Moriah Plaza Dead Sea Spa Hotel and the Carmel Forest Spa Resort, this bath helps to promote the elimination of acidic wastes from the body by encouraging perspiration. Excellent if you are suffering from muscular aches and pains and for warding off and treating colds and flu, it's a boon in the winter months.

100 g Dead Sea salts
4 drops tea tree essential oil
4 drops pine or cedar essential oil
6 drops patchouli oil

1 Add the Dead Sea salts to the bath while it is filling with comfortably hot water. Just before you step in, add the essential oils.
2 Drop a few drops of each essential oil into a warm, damp flannel or muslin cloth and place on your forehead. Soak for 20 minutes. Wrap up very warmly afterwards and sip a cup of soothing fennel or rosehip tea.

Deep heat boreh scrub

The perfect antidote to a chilly, wintry day or if you are feeling a cold or the flu coming on, this treatment is recommended by The Oberoi, Bali, Indonesia. Recognised as a traditional medicine, it is believed to help warm the body, relieve aching joints, sore muscles and headaches. It also increases blood circulation. Applied to the skin, it gives a wonderful all-over deep heat sensation. Avoid if you are pregnant or have very sensitive skin or conditions such as eczema.

1 tsp jojoba oil
4 tsp sandalwood powder
2 tsp ginger
2 tsp whole cloves
1 tsp cinnamon
1 tsp coriander seeds
1 tsp nutmeg
1 tsp turmeric
1 tsp black pepper
2 tsp rice powder
3 large carrots, grated finely

1 Mix the oil, herbs and spices and rice powder to make a thick paste. If you have a sensitive skin, use a larger amount of rice powder and reduce the amount of spices in the mix by half.
2 Cover your body with the paste and leave on for 5 to 10 minutes while you feel the warming sensation.
3 Massage it into your skin until it begins to slough off.
4 Follow by rubbing the carrot into your skin to moisturise.
5 Shower off and moisturise.

Mandi Kimiri dry skin booster

For post-holiday skin-that's-paper-dry, this intensive body smoother is more than a mere exfoliant. Your skin will feel incredibly soft and moist afterwards. Inspired by a recipe that's exclusive to The Jamu Traditional Spa, Bali, Indonesia, it smells so delicious, you'll want to eat it too.

50 g macadamia nuts
50 g peeled natural peanuts
1 tbsp freshly grated ginger
1 tbsp avocado or almond oil

1 Grind the nuts in a food processor, add the ginger and the oil and process until you get a crunchy peanut-butter style paste.
2 Rub the mixture over damp skin, massaging with firm, circular movements with the palms of your hands.
3 Rinse with warm water and pat your skin dry.

Tonic body rub

If you're feeling completely unrested after a night's sleep, try this stimulating body rub, inspired by treatments available at many French and Italian spas based on aromatic ingredients.

1 tbsp cider vinegar
5 drops lemon balm essential oil
5 drops tangerine essential oil
3 drops patchouli essential oil
3 drops juniper essential oil
2 drops rosemary essential oil
300 ml orange flower water

1 Add all the ingredients to a dark glass bottle and shake thoroughly to blend.
2 Have a warm shower and towel dry your skin vigorously.
3 While you are still standing in the tub or shower, sprinkle the essential oil tonic liberally on to your hands and apply all over your body, working from your feet upwards. Your skin will feel tingly, your mood uplifted and your energy levels will improve.

Therapeutic muscle fatigue bath

During a spa vacation, you may find that you've worked your body harder than ever before. Although this is one of the most enjoyable aspects of going to a spa, particularly if it is fitness orientated, like The Ashram, California or Canyon Ranch, Arizona, USA, you may find that your body aches and your muscles are fatigued after a day of hiking and cycling. Designed to help soothe away any aches, this therapeutic bath recipe is designed to relax and revitalise. Of course, it's just as useful after a day of gardening, a session at the gym or a long walk.

3 tbsp Epsom salts
2 drops marjoram essential oil
2 drops lavender essential oil
2 drops chamomile essential oil

1 Run a warm bath and add the Epsom salts. Swirl the water around to allow the salts to dissolve. Slip into the bath and add the essential oils.
2 Inhale the aroma deeply as you soak for about 20 minutes. Ensure that you keep warm after your bath.

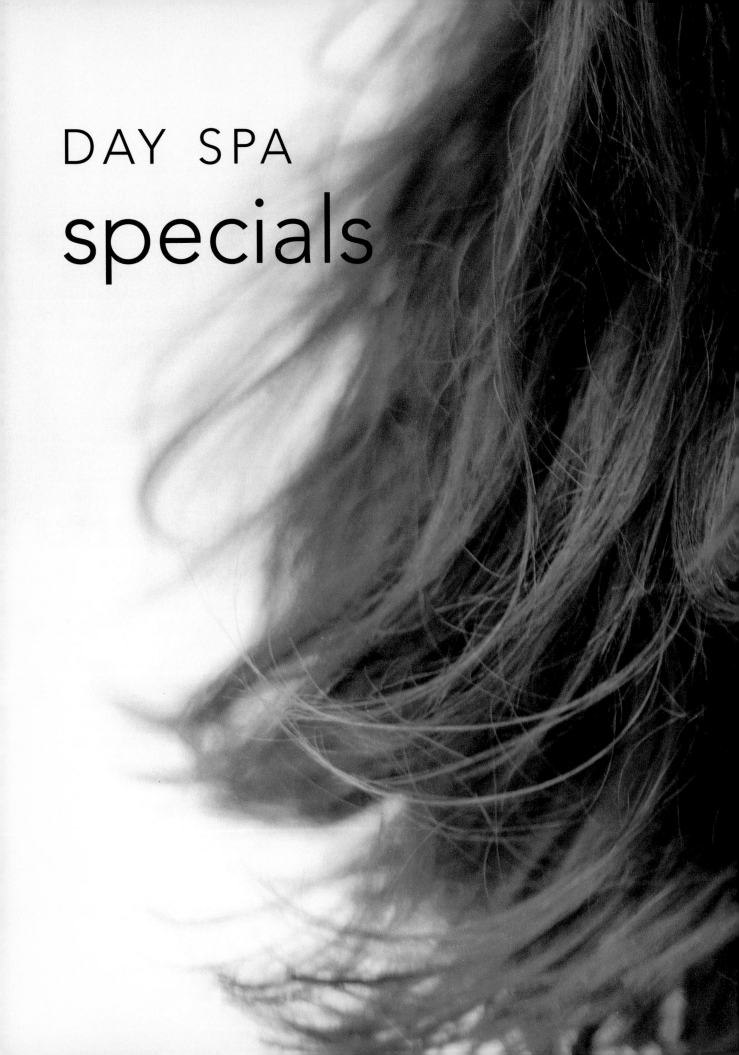

DAY SPA
specials

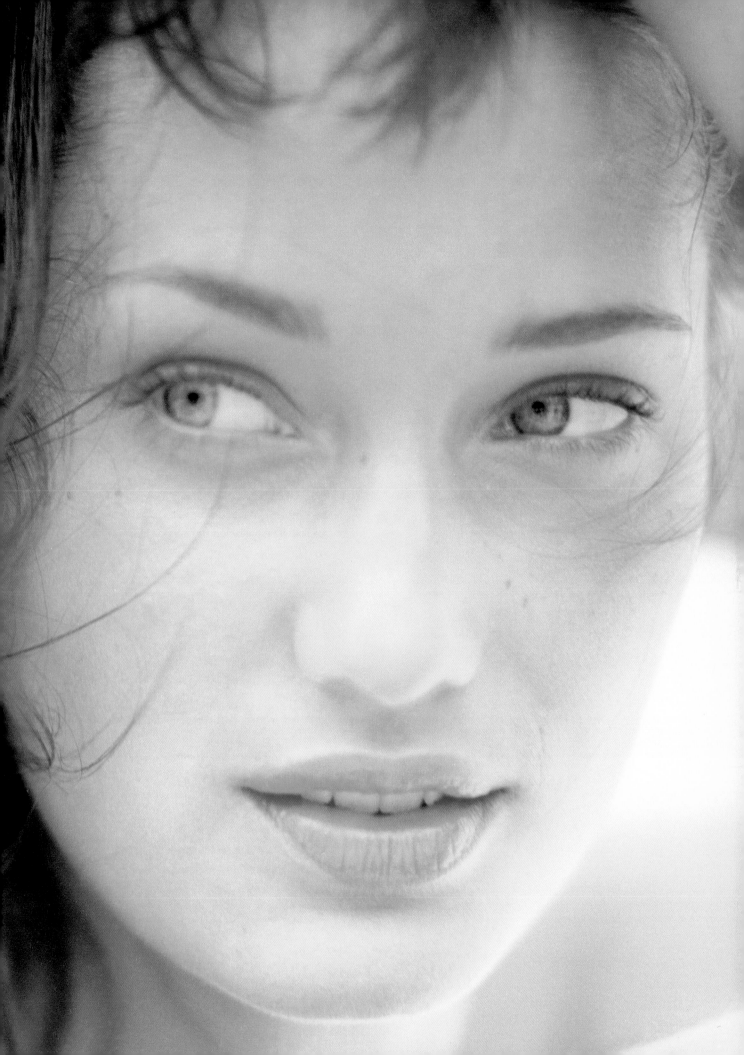

The chill-out day

When stress levels are soaring to an all-time high, dip into this soothing spa-it-at-home special, with tips and ideas from spas around the world.

DEEP BREATHING

Start your day with some deep breathing. Not only will it increase your energy levels, but it will also help to relax your mind and body.

• Sit on the floor with your legs crossed or on a chair that supports your back with your feet flat on the floor.

• Breathe in slowly, taking the breath through your nose. As you inhale, be conscious of the air passing along your windpipe, into your lungs and diaphragm. Focus on your breath as it travels down.

• Exhale slowly and steadily, ensuring that you are constantly focused on your breathing. Practise this cycle for about 5 minutes.

INSTANT CALMER

Run a warm bath and add to it this soothing bath oil combination from a recipe at the Nusa Dua Spa, Bali, Indonesia.

Tranquillity oil: 3 drops of vetiver essential oil, 3 drops of ylang ylang essential oil and 3 drops of sandalwood essential oil in 20 ml of soya or jojoba carrier oil.

As you soak in the water, try the Desert Healing Breath technique from Westward Look Resort, Arizona, USA, where guests are taught this calming deep-breathing exercise so that they can relax and recall the tranquillity of the desert after they return home.

• Close your eyes and picture the colours of the desert sky or a place that you love to visit. Imagine the warm wind blowing against your face and breathe deeply and slowly to the count of three.

• Absorb the fragrance of this place, hold it briefly, then gently release both your breath and any tension.

• Repeat several times, deepening your relaxation with each exhalation. By focusing on the sights and sounds and stimulations, you can cleanse your mind and spirit.

MEDICINE WALK

Dress in appropriate outdoor clothing and plan a leisurely walk in the park, along the beach or a nature reserve near your home. Try this Medicine Walk as experienced by guests at Vista Clara Ranch Resort and Spa, New Mexico, USA. Part of the Spa Ancestral Ways programme, it has been devised by Julie Rivers and Dona Wilder.

• Nurture yourself by taking a walk with a different point of view.

• In the Native American way, this could be called a Medicine Walk. Walk slowly, feeling your connection to the Earth Mother. Walk in awareness with soft eyes. Allow your eyes to gently scan your surroundings.

• If something catches your attention, such as a cloud, a bird or a stone in your path, take a moment to observe it more closely.

• Listen with soft ears. What is calling you? Is it the wind spirits, the song of the bird, the laughter of children or the flicker of butterfly wings? What is the message?

• Open your heart as you walk and follow your feelings – hug that tree, skip, dance or sing – responding to your inner urges. Be fully present in each moment of this walk, as you communicate with All Our Relations.

Calming cucumber and coconut mask

¼ unpeeled cucumber
1 tbsp almond milk (blend 2 tbsp almonds with
125 ml of water in a blender until smooth then
strain through a muslin cloth to extract the milk)
¼ avocado flesh
2 tbsp coconut oil
2 tbsp kaolin powder

1 Blend all the ingredients, apart from the kaolin,
in a blender until smooth.
2 Next, add the kaolin, little by little, to make a
paste that is firm but still workable.
3 Apply to your face with a pastry brush or your
fingertips and allow to dry for 10 to 15 minutes.
4 Rinse away with warm water. Pat your skin dry.

Complete the process by giving yourself a head
and face massage using a soothing blend of
essential oils. Try the Eastern serenity blend:
30 ml carrier oil, 3 drops patchouli essential oil,
2 drops sandalwood essential oil and 2 drops
jasmine essential oil; or the South-western
breeze: 30 ml carrier oil, 4 drops sage oil, 2 drops
cedarwood and 2 drops lavender essential oils.

Soothing herbal tea

Prepare yourself a soothing herbal tea. Try a
combination of hops, a natural sedative with
valerian, which is tension and anxiety reducing; or
blend a little passionflower with orange blossom,
both of which will help to induce restful sleep.
Prepare an infusion using 1 tbsp of each herb in
225 ml of boiling water. Strain and drink. Sweeten
with honey or add a little lemon juice to taste.

10-MINUTE SHIATSU-STYLE MASSAGE

Created by the experts at The Spa at St David's Hotel, Cardiff,
UK, treat yourself to a restorative shiatsu-style massage that will
not only restore a glow to your face, but will work at a deeper
level on the rest of the body.

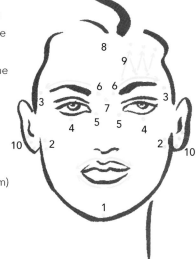

1 Use a downward
pressure and press three
times with the pad of one
finger on each hand to
stimulate the points in the
following way:
Start with the point
located in the centre of
the chin and work your
way through each point
from 1 to 10 (see diagram)
in sequence.

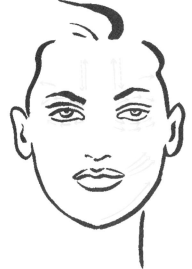

2 Repeat the sequence
two or three times.
3 Finish by using light,
sweeping finger
movements as indicated
by the arrow above to
stimulate lymphatic
drainage. Work towards
the temples, ears and jaw
line, as shown in the
diagram. This will help to
reduce puffiness and dark
circles around the eyes.

The wake-up call day

Feeling sluggish? In need of a some physical maintenance? Kick-start your energy levels and get your body into gear with this action-packed day. Try these muscle toning exercises recommended by the fitness experts at Lucknam Park, Wiltshire, UK.

Squats: stand up straight with your feet a shoulder-width apart. Bend your knees until your thighs are parallel to the ground. Keep your knees in line with your toes and over the ankles. Return to the starting position and repeat 10 to 15 times.

Lunges: stand up straight with your feet a shoulder-width apart. Take a big step forwards with one leg. Keep the knee just over the ankle and then bend your back leg so that the knee nearly touches the ground. Return the back knee so that it is straight, then bring back your front leg so that you return to a standing position. Repeat 10 to 15 times.

Sit-ups: lie down with your back flat on the ground. With your knees bent and arms out straight above your thighs, keep your chin up away from your chest. Raise your upper body until your fingertips touch or go past your knees, then return to starting position and do a further 10 to 15 repetitions.

Walk this way: one of the best ways to get fit and to maintain fitness is to Power Walk. Not only does it get you outside and away from your desk, housework and day-to-day anxieties, but it is incredibly easy to fit into a busy schedule. Plan to take a moderate to brisk paced walk of at least 30 minutes duration. (See pages 82-3 for a walking programme.)

POST-WORKOUT COOLER
Quench your thirst and refresh your palette with this low-calorie smoothie, a favourite of Leila Fazel, co-creator of Agua at Delano, Florida, USA, and Agua at Sanderson, London, UK. Combine 450 ml frozen honey dew melon, 2 tbsp fresh mint, 1 tbsp lime juice and 90 ml ginger ale with six ice cubes in a blender until slushy. Drink and relax, contemplating what you have just achieved.

Feet treat

If you've been busy working out, the chances are that your feet will be in need of some attention, no matter how supportive your training shoes are. Try these soothing foot remedies.

1 Massage your feet with sesame or olive oil and a few drops each of tea tree, eucalyptus and peppermint essential oils. This will help to soothe tired, hot feet and act as a natural deodorant.
2 If your feet are very callused, scrub them with a body scrub, rinse with warm water and cover with cocoa butter. Wrap your feet in plastic wrap and put on a pair of socks. Leave for at least an hour.
3 Give your feet a foot bath by adding a handful of fresh sage, lavender or bay and a tablespoon of sea salt to a basin of hot water. Soak your feet for at least 10 minutes.

Post-sports massage

When you have been working out, treat your body to a soothing, muscle-relaxing massage.

25 ml soya or avocado oil
10 drops marjoram essential oil
4 drops ginger essential oil
3 drops black pepper essential oil

1 Blend all the ingredients together in a dark glass bottle.
2 Pour a little in the palm of your hand to warm it up, then use smooth sweeping movements, working upwards and towards the heart to massage your feet, legs, buttocks, upper arms, shoulders and stomach.

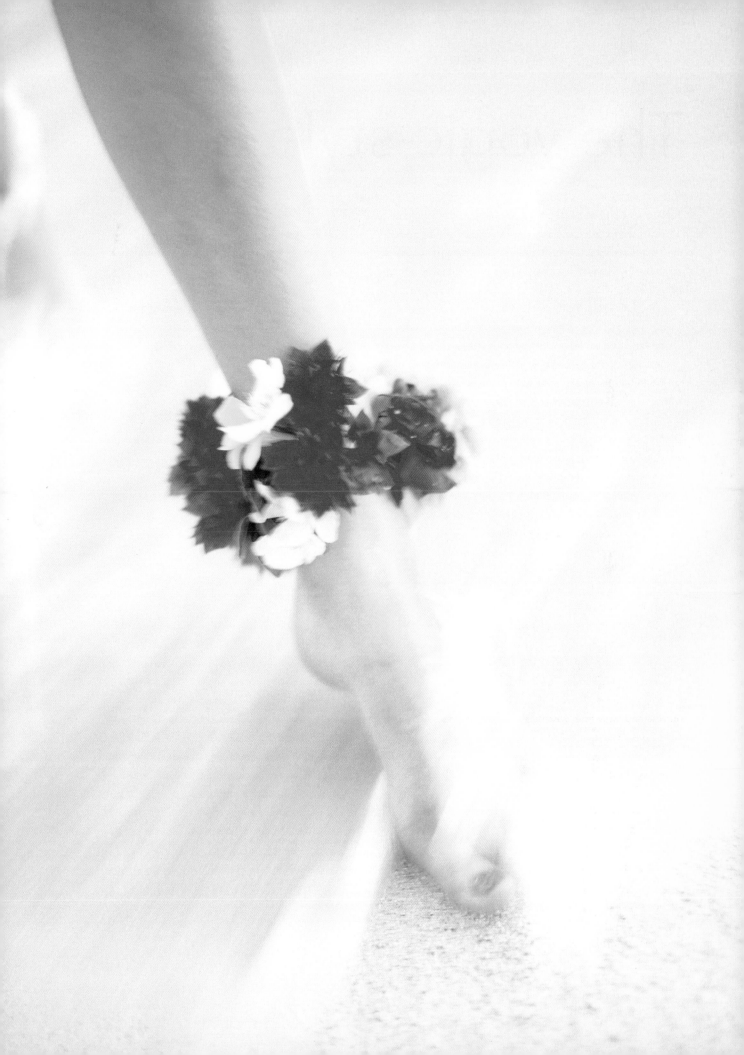

The yogic-style day

Many spas, East and West, now offer a wide range of ayurvedic and yogic therapies as part of their programmes. If you are feeling stuck in a rut and in need of a kick-start, try this yogic-style spa day.

THE YOGIC DIET

The yogic way of eating is based on ancient Indian teachings that suggest that all the energy in the universe, including food, has three qualities – inertia or darkness, known as tamas; purity, called sattva; and activity or passion – rajas. Tamasic foods, including fish, eggs, alcohol, vinegar, fried and barbecued foods, produce lethargy and a feeling of bloatedness when eaten in excess. Rajasic foods, such as garlic, onions, spiced and salted foods, soft drinks and chocolate, tea and coffee, can upset the balance of mind and body by over-stimulating the mind and making you feel restless and stressed. Sattvic foods, which include milk, butter, cheese, fresh and dried fruits, salads, grains, pulses, fresh herbs, nuts and seeds, are, on the other hand, calming and easy to digest. They also help to boost stamina and intellect. Try to ensure that you steer clear of rajasic and tamasic foods and boost your intake of sattvic foods.

Nourishing coconut rice and vegetables

Makes 2 servings

Try this very simple ayurvedic-style soup, designed to revitalise the mind, body and soul from The Taj Ayurvedic Centre at the Taj Residency, Kerala, India.

175 g rice
½ onion (about 50 g), peeled and sliced
1½ carrots (about 100 g), peeled and sliced
100 g baby corn, sliced
¼ head of broccoli (about 100 g), stalks removed and broken into florets
4 spring onions, green parts removed and white parts sliced thinly
75 ml coconut milk
salt
1 tsp chopped coriander, to garnish

1 Cook the rice in plenty of boiling salted water for approximately 15 minutes. Drain, retaining about 400 ml of the cooking water, and set aside the cooked rice.
2 Brown the onion in a non-stick pan.
3 Heat the rice water and add the carrots. Boil for approximately 5 minutes.
4 Add the corn, broccoli and spring onions to the pan with the carrots, along with the cooked onion, and cook for a further 5 to 10 minutes, until the vegetables are soft.
5 Reduce the heat and stir in the coconut milk. Do not re-heat the soup after adding the coconut milk or it will curdle. Season and garnish with a few spoonfuls of boiled rice and the chopped coriander.

Five-minute yoga sequence

Yoga not only helps to increase flexibility, it also boosts energy levels, relaxes the mind and improves digestion. Incorporate this yoga sequence, devised by Jennifer Fox and Paul Gould, fitness instructors from Rancho La Puerta, Baja California, Mexico, based on Iyengar yoga.

MOUNTAIN (TADASANA)

Stand evenly balanced on your feet. Pull up through your thighs. Maintaining the natural curves of your spine, try to stand as straight as possible. Imagine that you are a soaring mountain, centred and rising up strongly.

CHAIR (UTKATASANA)

Stretch your arms straight up, lower your thighs towards a parallel line with the ground. Keep your chest as far back as possible and breathe naturally through your nose. You are transforming rounded and stiff shoulders as you fully expand the chest for better posture and deeper breathing.

UPWARD DOG (URDHVAH MUKHA SVANASANA)

Pressing your palms into a low ledge or bench, bring your pelvis and base of spine forwards and lightly contract your buttocks. Work your legs back without bending or resting your knees. Keep your chest lifted and shoulders rolled back. You are opening the upper chest, strengthening the backs of your arms.

DOWNWARD DOG (ADHO MUKHA SVANASANA)

Make your knees firm, lift your hips and pull back your thighs for an invigorating stretch of the legs, shoulders and arms. Stay in the posture for between 15 seconds and 1 minute and breathe deeply. Repeat twice. The dog pose helps to reduce fatigue and boost energy.

Traditional Indian-style milk bath

Based on ancient Indian milk bath recipes, this will leave your skin smooth and your mind relaxed.

250 ml fresh milk
1 tsp oatmeal
2 drops rose essential oil

1 Mix the milk, oatmeal and rose essential oil together, then pour into a warm bath.
2 Relax in the bath for at least half an hour.

Traditional Indian-style body polish

This skin-buffing recipe is handed down from generation to generation by Indian women.

2 tbsp fresh milk
1 tbsp chick pea flour
pinch turmeric

1 Mix together all the ingredients.
2 Massage into damp skin to cleanse, buff and moisturise.

The aqua-therapy day

Water has long been associated with well-being and for many of us, an invigorating shower or relaxing bath is all the therapy we need when we are stressed out or feeling below par. Indulge in a day of water therapy to recharge your batteries and reduce stress levels.

HEALING HOT WATER
Ditch all caffeinated beverages, such as coffee and cola, and exchange them for water or herbal tisanes. For indigestion, try peppermint; for anxiety, headaches and water retention, try chamomile; for colds and flu, try cinnamon or nutmeg and to boost your mood, sip lemon balm.

DIP IN
One of the most therapeutic ways to keep fit, swimming not only tones muscles and increases aerobic fitness, but it is also incredibly relaxing. Aim to spend at least an hour in the pool, using a combination of different strokes to work on different parts of your body.
• Backstroke: good for shoulders and promoting relaxation.
• Breaststroke: excellent for toning upper arms and inner thighs.
• Butterfly: the best stroke for building stamina and for aerobic endurance.
• Crawl: a great aerobic workout, this stroke also tones the arms and works on the shoulders and upper back muscles.

WATER-TREADING
Many spas, particularly those in Austria, France and Germany, offer this hydrotherapy treatment as a cure for insomnia, nervous tension and to promote general well being. Fill your tub to mid-calf depth with cold water and add a few trays of ice cubes. Wrap your upper body in a warm, towelling robe and step into the bath. March on the spot so that one foot comes fully out of the water while the other stays submerged. Stay in for 1 minute initially and build up gradually until you are treading water for about 3 minutes. Afterwards, dry your feet and legs thoroughly , wrap up warmly and put on some cosy socks to sustain that feeling of relaxation.

Cleopatra dreamsicle bath
For a rejuvenating bathing experience, try this exotic recipe from Cindy 'Hilani' Woodward at the Golden Door, California, USA, guaranteed to turn your bath into Nirvana.

125 ml milk
1 sliced orange

1 Add the milk to a warm bath under a running tap.
2 Wrap the sliced orange in a muslin cloth and squeeze into the water to release the oil and juice.
3 Lie back and enjoy the heavenly aroma.

Eye bath
Refresh tired, computer-strained eyes with a soothing eye bath made with water and herbs.

500 ml water
10 ml dried eyebright or agrimony

1 Add the herbs to the water and boil for 20 minutes.
2 Strain and allow to cool, then pour into two tea cups and use to bathe each eye separately.
3 Soak two cotton pads in the water and use as compresses on your eyes.

Skin booster
While drinking at least eight glasses of water a day is the best way to ensure that skin hydration levels are maintained, this facial hydrotherapy treatment will tone and tighten skin. Use a hand-held shower and cool water to shower your face with a steady flow of water. Hold your head forwards over the bath and hold the shower as close to your face as is comfortable. Circle the shower around your face in a clockwise direction and repeat this three to five times before spraying anti-clockwise. Next, concentrate the spray on your forehead for 30 seconds, your temples and then your jawline. Pat your skin dry.

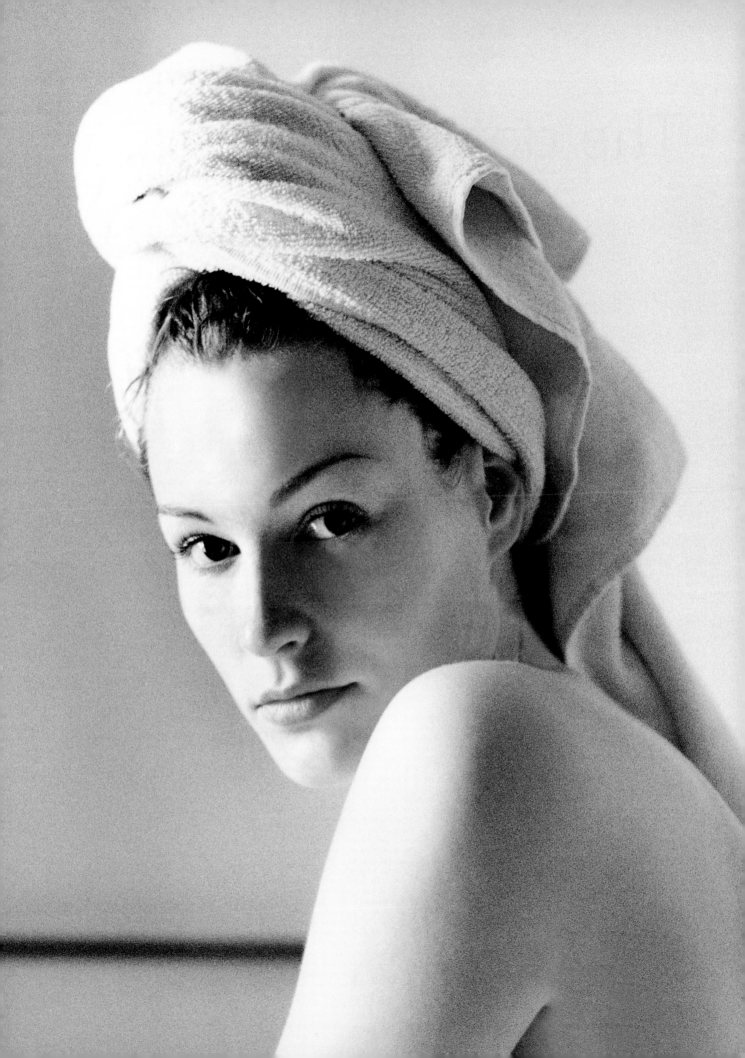

The detox day

If your energy levels are low, your skin and hair looking less than lustrous and you've been over-indulging of late, try a few of these cleansing treats.

DETOX DRINKS

Start the day with a cleansing drink. Squeeze the juice of half a lemon into a cup of freshly boiled water or into freshly squeezed orange juice and sip. Alternatively, brew up some peppermint, elderflower, yarrow or wild thyme tea, all of which will help your body to dispose of toxins, such as alcohol.

CLEANSING FOODS

If you are following a detox programme, even if it's just for the day look to the following points:
• Cut down on red meat, refined sugar, pasta, bread and rice, alcohol, coffee and caffeinated beverages such as cola, crisps, biscuits, pre-packaged and convenience foods.
• Instead, stockpile low-toxin foods such as corn, salmon, brown rice, sardines and organic chicken and turkey.
• Increase your intake of fresh fruits such as apricots, blueberries, raspberries, oranges, apples and papaya and cleansing vegetables including tomatoes, broccoli, Brussels sprouts, spinach, beetroot and celery.
• Drink at least 2 litres of filtered or bottled water while you are detoxing.
• Take 1000 mg of antioxidant rich vitamin C to help cleanse and revitalise your system.

Clearing your head

If your hair and scalp are in need of some deep cleansing and detoxing, try this intensive treatment, based on a recipe from The Spa at The Bali Hyatt, Bali, Indonesia.

15 ml macadamia or coconut oil
10 drops eucalyptus, rosemary, cedarwood or tea tree essential oils
1 mashed avocado
2 tbsp cider vinegar

1 Warm the macadamia or coconut oil in a bain-marie or in an oil burner and add the essential oil of your choice.
2 Apply the warm oil to the roots of your hair and massage down the hair shaft, working towards the ends. Spend a few minutes massaging your scalp with firm, circular movements of your fingertips. Work from the nape of your neck to your crown and then to your forehead.
3 Once your hair is covered with the oil, apply the mashed avocado, concentrating on the ends rather than the scalp.
4 Wrap your head in a hot towel or wear a plastic shower cap.
5 Leave on for 10 to 15 minutes, and then rinse thoroughly with warm water. Shampoo once or twice, rinse again then pour on the cider vinegar as a final rinse.

Thai mud wrap

Body wraps are renowned for their detoxifying abilities, drawing impurities out of the skin. Try this recipe based on a secret mud mix from The Oriental Spa at The Oriental, Bangkok, Thailand.

125 ml green clay or kaolin
125 ml organic milk
125 ml sesame oil
½ tsp turmeric powder
½ tsp sandalwood powder

1 Blend all the ingredients until a paste is formed.
2 Slather on to your body and wrap yourself in a plastic sheet (a foil survival sheet from camping shops is ideal) and then in several large, warm bath sheet towels.
3 Keep warm for 20 minutes, then unwrap yourself and rinse the mask away with warm water.

Salty solution

Try this traditional old-style spa salt bath for a deep-cleansing experience. Run a warm bath and add 150 g of Epsom salts, 4 drops of sage and 2 drops of tea tree essential oils. Lie back, head on a rolled-up towel and steep your body, ensuring that the water level comes right up to your neck. Keep the water as hot as is comfortable and relax for about 25 minutes. Slip straight into bed afterwards and ensure that you keep your body warm with a hot-water bottle and some cosy pyjamas and socks. Remember to drink lots of water, as your body will lose fluid via perspiration.

Juice it

If you are planning a detox day, incorporate plenty of fresh vegetable and fruit juices into your programme. Not only are they excellent sources of vitamins, minerals and fibre, they are also brilliant detoxifiers. To get the full benefits of fresh juices, you need to drink them as soon as they are blended. You can stick to separate vegetable or fruit combinations or blend fruits and vegetables to increase their therapeutic benefits. Try these combinations:
Fruits: grapefruit, orange and lemon; apple and cranberry; orange, papaya and melon.
Vegetables: celery, carrot and beetroot; tomato and celery; celery, lettuce and spinach.
Mixed fruit and vegetables: apple, celery and fresh root ginger; carrot and pear; carrot, orange, apple and lemon; beetroot and carrot.

Salt and soya oil scrub

Stimulate your circulation and slough away dead skin cells with an salt and soya oil body scrub.

100 g sea salt
125 ml soya oil
3 drops sage or eucalyptus essential oil

1 Blend all the ingredients roughly in a bowl.
2 Dampen your skin under the shower. Then grab a handful of the salt and oil mixture and massage into your skin, working from your ankles upwards.
3 Finish with a short spritz of cold water, then back to warm water to rinse the body scrub away.

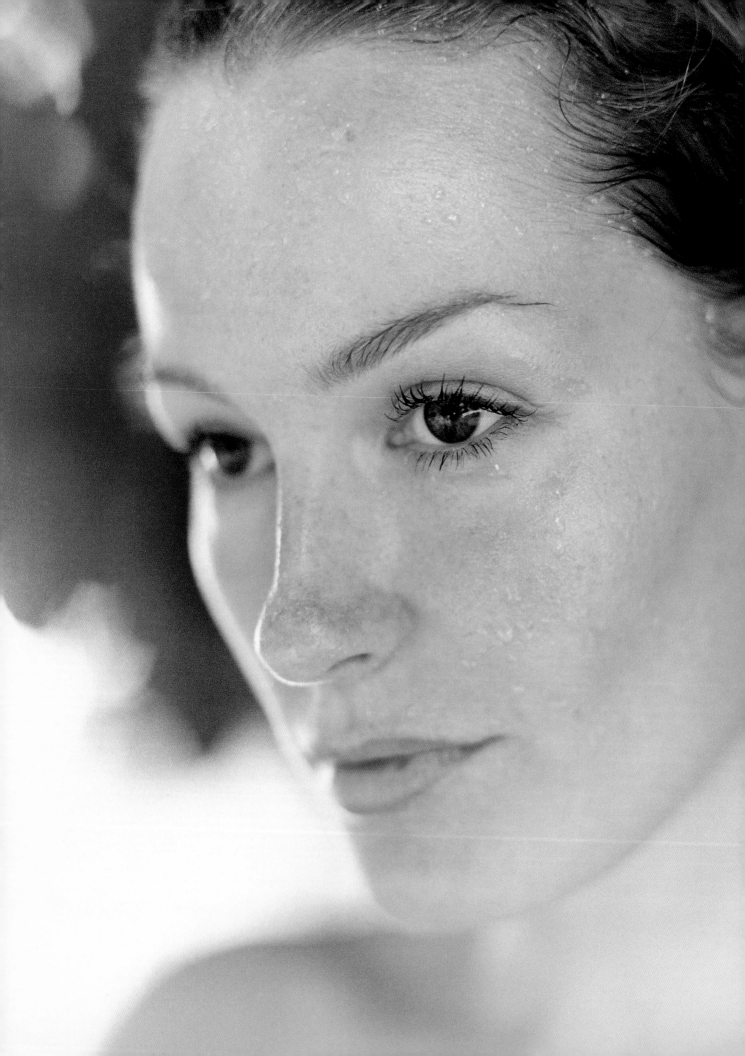

Spa Directory

Spas are as individual as you are – some are great all-rounders while others are best for fitness, pampering or simply chilling out. With this in mind, we've created this back-to-basics, at-a-glance guide to give you a helping hand when you're booking your much deserved spa break. There are, quite literally, hundreds of spas throughout the world. This is a selection of some of my personal favourites and those considered to be the best in their particular field. For other spa listings, consult the following:

Spatours
Website:
members.aol.com/spatours/spas.htm
SpaAsia
Website: www.spaasia.com
Spa Finder
Website: www.spafinder.com
Tel: +1 212 924 6800

AUSTRALIA

Azabu
End of Skinners Shoot Road
Byron Bay
NSW 2481
Australia
Tel: +61 2 6680 9102
Fax: + 61 2 6680 9103
Website: www.azabu.com.au
Anyone who yearns for respite from the modern world will adore Azabu, a private, tropical-style spa located in 5 acres of tropical native forest. There are only five suites, all with their own private balconies and sunken spa tubs. Aveda treatments are available at Azabu's Aveda Day Spa. For the ultimate in luxurious pampering, peace and quiet, Azabu is a must.

The Cape Retreat
PO Box 810
Byron Bay

New South Wales 2481
Australia
Tel: +61 2 6684 1363
Fax: +61 2 6684 3461
Email: caperet@om.com.au
Website: www.bayweb.com.au/caperetreat
Located in the scenic area of Byron Bay, Cape Retreat is situated in 120 acres of rainforest on one side and beautiful, unspoiled beaches on the other. A wide selection of outdoor activities including Bush walking, cycling along the beach, fishing and outdoor massage are on the menu and accommodation is in Tandy's Cottage, a small colonial style house. This very relaxed, chill-out type of resort will suit those who want to escape from the crowds.

Couran Cove Resort Spa and Total Living Centre
PO Box 224
Runaway Bay
Queensland 4216
Australia
Tel: +61 7 5597 9000
Fax: +61 2 5597 9090
E-mail: enquiry@couran-cove.com.au
Website: www.couran-cove.com.au
Located just a few miles from Australia's heavenly Gold Coast, Couran Cove Resort is nestled on South Stradbroke Island. Outdoor sports are a speciality here, with a dazzling choice of basketball, kayaking and rock climbing, to name but a few of the activities. Accommodation is in one of the beautifully designed eco-cabins, villas and lodges with their own private decks overlooking the lagoon or forest. For pampering, the Spa Island has an Olympic-sized swimming pool, massage huts and t'ai chi classes.

Daintree Eco-Lodge and Spa
20 Daintree Road
Daintree
Queensland 4873
Australia
Tel: +61 7 4098 6100
Fax: +61 7 4098 6200
E-mail: info@daintree-ecolodge.com.au
Website: www.daintree-ecolodge.com.au

Set in the world's oldest living rainforest – the 110 million year old Daintree – and located metres away from the majestic Daintree River, the Lodge offers the quintessential tropical experience. The 30 acre site is an ecological time capsule where guests experience close encounters with primeval plants, indigenous folklore, gourmet cuisine, luxury accommodation in tree house villas and the latest in health and relaxation treatments. Daintree offers a wide menu of beauty and body treatments.

Eaglereach Wilderness Resort
Summer Hill Road
Vacy NSW 2421
Australia
Tel: +61 2 4938 8233
Fax: +61 2 4938 8234
E-mail: enquiry@eaglereach.com.au
Website: www.eaglereach.com.au
For those who want to escape to the wilderness, Eagle Reach is just the ticket. Situated above Barrington Tops, one of Australia's largest National Parks and with views of the Pacific Ocean, accommodation is in one of 36 luxury lodges. Activities range from swimming and Bush walking to fishing and riding with plenty of fresh health-conscious food and nurturing treatments thrown in.

Empire Retreat
Caves Road
Yallingup
Western Australia 6282
Australia
Tel: +61 8 9755 2065
Fax: +61 8 9755 2297
E-mail: empire@compwest.net.au
Website: www.empireretreat.com.au
Set on a working farm with a lake in 265 acres in Western Australia's wine region, the Empire Retreat offers luxury and seclusion. Soothing interiors created with natural wood and stone with interconnecting outdoor wooden boardwalks make this a unique environment. Enjoy a wide range of outdoor activities including Bush walking, fishing and cycling and a full menu of pampering beauty treats.

The Golden Door Health Retreat

Ruffles Road
Willow Vale
Queensland 4209
Australia
Tel: +61 7 5546 6855 Fax: +61 7 5546 6173
E-mail: golddoor@othenet.com.au
Website: www.goldendoor.com.au
If changing your lifestyle is your goal, The Golden Door is well worth a visit. Renowned for its well-rounded spa programme, there is everything from yoga to feldenkrais bodywork on offer, all in breathtakingly beautiful surroundings.

Hyatt Regency-Coolum

PO Box 78
Coolum Beach
Queensland 4573
Australia
Tel: +61 754 461 234
Fax: +61 7544 62957
E-mail: coolum@hyatt.com.au
Website: www.hyatt.com
Located slap-dash in between the Pacific and the rainforests and bush lands of Mt Coolum National Park, the Hyatt Regency-Coolum sits on Australia's Sunshine Coast. The state-of-the-art spa and fitness centre offers everything from aerobics to yoga, hiking to riding together with a complete menu of face and body treats.

The Observatory Hotel Spa

89-113 Kent Street
Sydney 2000
Australia
Tel: +61 2 9256 2229
Fax: +61 2 9256 2235
E-mail: observatory@mail.com
Website: www.observatoryhotel.com.au
Stay in five-star luxury at the Observatory Hotel and slip in to its equally luxurious Day Spa Health and Leisure Club to experience treatments as varied as hydrotherapy, shirodarah – an ayurvedic ritual hot oil treatment and – massage. The spa also offers a state-of-the-art health club with a 20 metre heated pool and a Dead Sea salt flotation tank, steam room, dry sauna and Jacuzzi.

The Sanctuary Holistic Retreat

PO Box 270
Bangalow
New South Wales 2479
Australia
Tel: +61 2 6687 1216

Fax : +61 2 6687 1310
Website: www.sanctuary.org.au
Set in the lush environment of Byron Bay, this holistic retreat offers vegetarian cuisine, holistic workshops, chi gung, meditation, yoga, tennis, volleyball and a gorgeous lap pool. The emphasis is on mind, body and spirit at this nurturing spa.

Shizuka Ryokan

8 Lakeside Drive
Hepburn Springs
Victoria 3461
Australia
Tel: +61 3 5348 2030
Fax: +61 3 5348 1358
Website : www.shizuka.com.au
A very special spa, the Shizuka Ryokan is built in the style of an ancient Japanese-style inn (Ryokan). Nestled among huge pine trees, it is perfect for couples and small groups as there are only seven rooms. In-your-own-room shiatsu and aromatherapy treatments mean that you can just roll into bed for the best night's sleep ever.

Solar Springs Health Retreat

96 Osborn Avenue
Bundanoon
New South Wales 2578
Australia
Tel: +61 2 4883 6027
Fax: +61 2 4862 1809
E-mail : enquire@solar.com.au
Website : www.solar.com.au
From cycling, archery, t'ai chi, yoga and Bush walking to reiki, massage and bowen therapy – a treatment involving gentle stimulation of energy flow in the body – Solar Springs is a holistic retreat offering a selection of accommodation that ranges from deluxe to simple. Luxurious facials, body wrap, peels and baths and mainly vegetarian food complete the package and leave you feeling refreshed and renewed.

CANADA

Echo Valley Ranch Resort

Clinton
Jesmond BC
Canada
Tel: +1 250 459 2386
E-mail: evranch@uniserve.com
If you long for space and sanctuary, Echo Valley Ranch Resort, located in the Canadian

wilderness, a family run spa for only 20 guests at a time, could be the place for you. With lodge-style and log cabin accommodation, the feeling is rustic and cosy. Take a hike across an Indian Reservation and sleep under the stars in your own personal tepee, or partake in some river rafting or bird watching. Luxurious spa treatments, from aromatherapy to hydrotherapy, will ease any muscle fatigue after your day in the wild. The perfect stop-off for anyone who has always wanted to be a bit of a pioneer but likes a dose of luxury to boot.

Mountain Trek Fitness Retreat and Health Spa

PO Box 1352
Ainsworth Hot Springs
British Columbia V0G 1AO
Canada
Tel: +1 250 229 5636
Fax: +1 250 229 5246
Website: www.hiking.com
Set in the beautiful surroundings of the Kootenay Mountains, British Columbia, this spa offers hiking heaven. With only 13 guests at a time, you're guaranteed personal attention at all times, especially on the long and sometimes arduous hikes across the spectacular mountain range. The hearty vegetarian menu, high in complex carbohydrates and low in fat, will ensure that you return home fitter, firmer and toxin free. And for those who want a sprinkling of pampering with hiking, massage, hydrotherapy and an array of pampering treats are available. Other activities include yoga, golf, cycling and skiing.

Solace Spa at Banff Springs Hotel

Alberta
Canada
Tel: +1 403 762 2211
Fax: +1 403 762 5755
E-mail: res.vshres@vsh.dphotels.ca
Website: www.fairmont.com
This castle-like hotel in the Canadian Rockies is reminiscent of the hotel in The Shining, but don't let that put you off. The spa menu includes body wraps, scrubs, mineral and herbal baths and aromatherapy massage. Fitness activities include aerobics, skiing, sailing, riding, golf, tennis and cycling. The breathtaking and clear mountain air will leave you feeling invigorated while the luxurious service is certain to leave you feeling totally spoiled.

THE CARIBBEAN

La Casa de Vida Natural
Rio Grande
Puerto Rico
Tel: +1 787 887 4359
La Casa is a unique health retreat that will appeal to those searching for enlightenment and an antidote to a stressful lifestyle that they can also take back home. Weekend getaways and five night workshops are on offer with a variety of activities including aerobics, yoga and meditation, hiking, water sports and t'ai chi. Accommodation is simple but comfortable and you will definitely check out feeling rejuvenated and revived.

Le Sport
Gros Islet
St Lucia
Tel: +1 758 450 8551
Fax: +1 758 450 0368
E-mail: lesport@candw.lc
A great escape for those looking for the pleasures of a traditional beach holiday with sun, sand and surf combined with the latest in health, fitness and beauty. Every activity from windsurfing and tennis to cycling and scuba diving can be found here. Escape to the Moorish-style Oasis-spa for delicious salt-scrub body rubs, revitalising hydrotherapy and meltingly relaxing massages.

FRANCE

Caudalie Institut de Vinotherapie
Les Sources de Caudalie
Chemin de Smith Haut-Lafitte
33650 Martillac
France
Tel: +33 5 57 83 82 82
Fax: +33 5 57 83 82 81
E-mail: Sources@sources-caudalie.com
Website: www.sources-caudalie.com
Nestling beside Les Sources de Caudalie hotel and restaurant in a beautiful vineyard, the Caudalie spa offers a unique range of health and beauty cures combining the benefits of hot spring water, grape and vine extracts. From the red vine bath and merlot wraps to the barrel bath and underwater exhilarating shower, you won't find these treatments anywhere else on earth. The spa's programme also includes herbal tea infusions, grape drinks and a detox course, based – no surprises here – on grapes.

Domaine du Royal Club Evian
Hotel Royal
Rive Suid de Lac de Geneva
74500 Evian-Les-Bains
France
Tel: +33 4 50 26 85 00
The spa at Evian, the source of the famous mineral water, is one of the best hydrotherapy centres in the world. Every guest undergoes a medical examination to determine the cure that would best suit their needs and then prescribed a treatment regime. From ozone and oxygen baths to underwater massage and Turkish baths, there is, quite literally, every water treatment under the sun. For those who want activity, there is an extensive menu of sport and fitness activities.

Institute of Thalassotherapy Louison Bobet
Hotel Miramar
13 Rue Louison Bobet
64200 Biarritz
France
Tel: + 33 5 59 41 30 00
Set on the Atlantic coast in the beautiful resort of Biarritz, the Institute of Thalassotherapy is one of France's foremost seawater and seaweed treatment centres. From jet showers, multi-jet baths, seaweed body masks, a heated seawater swimming pool and an extensive range of fitness and aqua aerobics classes, you'll find a plethora of therapeutic seaweed and seawater activities. Outdoor activities including riding, tennis and seasonal skiing are all available too.

GERMANY

Brenner's Park Hotel
Sehiller Strasse 4-6
76530 Baden-Baden
Germany
Tel: +49 72 21 9000
E-mail: reservations@brenners-park.de
Website: www.brenners-park.de
Located on the edge of the Black Forest, the Brenner's Park Hotel houses the world-famous Lancaster Beauty Farm, for the ultimate in top-to-toe pampering. Bathe in the healing waters of the Roman-style baths, partake of the gorgeous five-star Lancaster menu of beauty treatments, take a yoga class or, if you're after more active, outdoor pursuits, there's hiking, golf, tennis, seasonal cross country skiing, riding and cycling.

INDIA

The Kairali Ayurvedic Health Resort
Palakkad
Kodumbu
Palakkad District 678551
Kerala
India
Tel: +91 492 322553
Fax :+91 492 322732
E-mail:kairali@giasdl01.vsnl.net.in
Website: www.kairali.com
A resort with a difference, Kairali is set amidst 50 acres of tropical greenery in Palakkad, Kerala, known as God's Own Country. Dedicated to bringing you the science of ayurvedic health care, the menu includes traditional oil massages, yoga and meditation together with a variety of special Ayurvedic cures for ailments as varied as arthritis, migraine, stress and fatigue.

The Spa at Rajvilas
Rajvilas Hotel
Goner Road
Jaipur 303 012
India
Tel: +91 141 64 0101
Fax: +91 141 64 0202
Like all Oberoi hotels, the Rajvilas is luxury incarnate. Set in 32 acres of lush gardens, accommodation is deluxe with a capital 'D', many of the rooms having their own pool, luxury tents and outdoor deck. With its palatial interior, all rooms have enormous four-poster beds and sunken marble baths overlooking private walled gardens. The spa itself offers deluxe service with a full menu of holistic, ayurvedic and traditional Western relaxation and beauty treatments. If you want to feel and look like a princess, then The Spa at Rajvilas is the destination for you.

The Taj Ayurvedic Centre
Taj Residency
Calicut
Kerala
India
Tel: + 91 492 239939
This is one of India's most respected ayurvedic centres, offering in-depth cures and programmes to treat a wide range of ailments. From abhyanga, where oil is used in gentle massage to help reduce fatigue, improve sleep and delay ageing, to snana, a bath with herbal powders and dhara, in which medicated oil, milk or buttermilk are poured

onto your head in a continuous stream, a comprehensive selection of treatments are carried out by respected ayurvedic practitioners. Yoga and meditation are also incorporated in the regimes, alongside specially created ayurvedic food to nourish mind, body and spirit.

INDONESIA

The Banyan Tree
Bintan Island
Site A4
Lagoi
Bintan Island
Indonesia
Tel: +62 7632 4374
Fax: +62 7718 1348
E-mail: bintan@banyantree.com
Built in traditional Indonesian-style, the Banyan Tree Spa is a hidden-away oasis overlooking the ocean that offers tranquillity in a tropical, lush paradise. Delicious pampering awaits you at the spa pavilion, where local ingredients and traditional recipes are used to scrub, soothe, nurture and rejuvenate from top-to-toe. Golf, windsurfing, sailing and snorkelling are just a few of the main activities at the Banyan.

Jamu Traditional Spa
KulKulBali
PO Box 3097
Denpasar
80030 Bali
Indonesia
Tel: +62 361 752520
Fax: +62 361 752519
For authentic Indonesian spa treatments without Western fluffiness, Jamu is the place. This is where you'll find luxurious, unique, all-natural skin treats like Mandi Kemiri and Jamu Tropical Nuts Facial, both based on folklore beauty remedies handed down from generation to generation.

The Jimbaran Spa at The Four Seasons Resort
Jimbaran Bay
Jimbaran
Denpasar 80361
Bali
Indonesia
Tel: +62 361 701010
Fax: +62 361 701020
E-mail: Belinda.Shepherd@fourseasons.com

One of the world's most beautiful and luxurious spas, The Spa at Jimbaran is an exotic, tropical retreat where five-star service combines with the natural Balinese ambience. The facilities are superb and the location breath-taking with indoor and outdoor private treatment rooms where you can shower in the midst of nature without inhibition. The food is a blend of traditional Indonesian mixed with the best in global cuisine with the emphasis on fresh, fragrant ingredients.

The Mandara Spa at The Chedi
Desa Melinggih Kelod Payangan
Gianyar 80572
Bali
Indonesia
Tel: +62 361 975963
Fax: +62 361 975963
E-mail: chediubd@ghmhotels.com
Website: www.ghmhotels.com
The Mandara Spa at The Chedi lies in the hills of Ubud, famous for its hippy hangouts. With an array of delicious treatments, The Mandara is famed for its floral bath, filled with hundreds of flower petals, and a special massage using five different techniques and performed by two therapists. Sheer Bliss. The food is Indonesian haute cuisine with a bias towards healthy ingredients and beautiful presentation. Definitely a place to retreat to if you are burnt out.

The Mandara Spa at The Ibah
Tjampuhan
Ubud
Bali
Indonesia
Tel: +62 361 974466
Fax: +62 361 974 467
E-mail: ibah@denpasar.wasantara.net.id
This family-run hotel and spa has a cosy feel, with only 11 individual rooms. The spa itself has a cocooning atmosphere with its traditional Balinese decor – teak wood and colonial-style furniture – and its wonderful private Jacuzzi pools. Exotic treatments, from the Bali kopi scrub coffee body polish to the exclusive Mandara massage that includes six massage styles including Hawaiian lomi-lomi, Swedish, Balinese, Shiatsu, Thai and aromatherapy, guarantee top-to-toe relaxation and rejuvenation.

Nusa Dua Beach Hotel and Spa
PO Box 1028
Denpasar

Bali
Indonesia
Tel: +62 361 771210
Fax: +62 361 772621
E-mail: ndbhnet@indosat.net.id
The epitome of luxury, the Nusa Dua Beach Hotel and Spa was built by the Sultan of Brunei with no expense spared. The spa has a beautiful lap pool surrounded by outdoor pavillions where the treatments are carried out and the decor is a blend of traditional Balinese dark wood, vivid painted walls and ikat and batik fabrics. Treatments are based on Balinese therapies with a huge menu of massages, rubs, baths and head, foot and face manipulation, many using local herbs and ingredients.

The Oberoi, Bali
Legian Beach
Jalan Kayu Aya
PO Box 3351
Denpasar 80001
Bali
Indonesia
Tel: +62 36 170361
Fax : +62 36 1730791
For reservations: 0800 962 096
Website: http://www.oberoihotels.com
Like its sister in Lombok, The Oberoi Bali offers luxurious treatments in wonderful, tranquil surroundings. The comprehensive spa menu includes a huge range of world class face and body treatments and some very unique traditional Indonesian indulgences like the Lalur too.

The Oberoi, Lombok
Medana Beach Tanjung
Mataram 83001 NTB
Lombok
Indonesia
Tel: +62 370 638 444
Fax: +62 370 632 496
For reservations: 0800 962 096
The Oberoi is unsurpassed in terms of architecture and the surroundings – there is nothing to touch it in Lombok for style and luxury. The treatments include everything from shiatsu to classical Swedish massage, and most interestingly, the Mandi Lulur, which is a traditional Javanese ceremony given to a woman by her friends each day during the week of her wedding, involving massage, herbal exfoliation and yoghurt splash, followed by a warm tropical flower filled aromatic soak in a sunken marble bath.

Spa at The Bali Hyatt

PO Box 392
Sanur
Bali
Indonesia
Tel: +62 361 281234
Fax: +62 361 287693
E-mail: bhyatt@dps.mega.net.id
Website: www.hyatt.com

Designed in the style of a Balinese village, Spa at the Bali Hyatt offers traditional Indonesian beauty with world class service. Partake of the sumptuous treatments in a private spa villa with its own sunken bath, outdoor shower and daybed. Experience a floral foot soak with every treatment, delicious skin-reviving body scrubs and hot oil scalp massages all in the tropical bougainvillea drenched environment. You'll be close to heaven.

ISRAEL

Carmel Forest Spa Resort

POB 90000
Haifa 31900
Israel
Tel: +972 4 8307888
Fax: +972 4 8323988
E-mail: carmelf@isrotel.co.il
Website: www.isrotel.co.il

Nestled in the green forests of Mount Carmel, the spa overlooks the sparkling waters of the Mediterranean. From an authentic Turkish hammam to t'ai chi lessons or meditation sessions, there is an atmosphere of blissful calm. Mud treatments are a speciality, as are the seasonal body wraps. For massage sophisticates, there are nine techniques to sample, from reiki to Thai. For the active, hiking, riding and mountain biking ensure you can be on the move from dawn until dusk.

Radisson Moriah Plaza Dead Sea Spa Hotel

Israel
Tel: +972 7 659 1591
Fax: +972 7 658 4238

For therapeutic Dead Sea hydrotherapy treatments, including mud wraps, sulphur-rich baths and underwater massage, The Spa at The Moriah Plaza offers an unrivalled treatment menu. Set on its own private beach, the spa also offers a variety of fitness activities including tennis, aerobics, swimming and basketball.

ITALY

Palazzo Arzaga Spa

25080 Carzago di Calvagese della Riviera
Brescia
Italy
Tel: +39 030 68 06 00
Fax: +39 030 68 06 168
E-mail: info@palazzoargaza.it

This fifteenth-century palace on the shores of Lake Garda houses the celebrated Argaza Spa, with its speciality being the Terme di Saturnia Spa face and body treatments from Tuscany. Unless you're into golf, this is very much a pampering and relaxing experience.

MALAYSIA

The Mandara Spa at The Datai

Jalan Telek Datai
07000 Palau Langkawi
Kedah Darul Aman
Malaysia
Tel: +60 4 9592500
Fax: +60 4 9592600

Located in the jungle, The Mandara Spa at The Datai offers a back-to-nature spa experience with plenty of luxury thrown in. Treatments are given in spa suites dotted along a stream. Try out the deluxe oriental massage or an outdoor stream bath in a rainforest environment to achieve a true sense of peace and calm.

MEXICO

Punta Serena

Km. 20 Carretera Federal 200
Tenacatita-Municipio de la Huerta
48989 Jalisco
Mexico
Tel: +52 335 15020/15100
Fax: +52 333 515050

Punta Serena calls itself a holistic retreat – and that's just what it is. Balanced high on a mountain overlooking Tenacatita Bay, it's a haven of natural beauty and tranquillity. Spiritual awareness programmes incorporating t'ai chi, yoga, chi kung and chakra work are on offer alongside fitness programmes, shamanism, reiki massage, a Native Mexican sweat lodge, tennis and riding. A place to leave your stress behind and learn new techniques to bring home at the end of your stay.

Rancho La Puerta

Tecate
Baja California
Mexico
Tel: +1 760 744 4222
Website: www.rancholapuerta.com

Rancho La Puerta rests at the foot of Mount Kuchumaa, sacred to the Kumeyaay Indians. Accommodation is in individual casitas, scattered around the 3000 acres of grounds. The ethos of the spa rests firmly in its roots – it was founded over 50 years ago by Edmond and Deborah Szekely and was the world's first fitness spa. With six tennis courts, six aerobic gyms, three swimming pools, five whirlpool-jet therapy pools and three saunas, every aspect of fitness is well catered for, while separate men and women's spas ensure that every part of your body is massaged, pampered and steamed to perfection. Yoga and meditation classes are also offered, together with the Inner Journey programme that caters for mind, body and spirit. The delicious food is a mixture of influences – you'll enjoy every morsel.

The Spa at Las Ventanas al Paradiso

Los Cabos
Mexico
Tel: +52 114 40300
For reservations: +44 (0)20 7333 7013

The Spa at Las Ventanas al Paraiso, one of Mexico's most beautiful hotels, is a cosy sanctuary offering a wonderful melange of treatments gathered from around the world, together with some that are unique to the spa and to this part of Mexico. Try la stone therapy, where hot, oiled stones are placed under and on your body, leaving you with a wonderful sense of calm, or simply float your troubles away under the stars in one of the outdoor hot tubs. Heavenly. Accommodation in Las Ventanas is in beautiful individual casitas that overlook the Pacific Ocean. Telescopes are provided for star gazing and whale watching and each casita has its own hot tub on a private deck.

SWITZERLAND

The Grand Hotel and Spa Victoria-Jungfrau

Hoheveg 41
3800 Interlaken
Switzerland
Tel: +41 33 828 28 28

E-mail: interlaken@victoria-jungfrau.ch
Website: www.victoria-jungfrau.ch
This stunning 19th-century hotel was completely restored recently with the addition of a state-of-the-art spa, making it one of Switzerland's most popular five-star retreats. The spa has a wonderful Roman-style pool, a saltwater bath, Turkish steam bath, Finnish sauna, medical check-ups and fitness assessments, together with a health-conscious menu and a plethora of restorative beauty treatments and massage therapies. Being adjacent to the Swiss Alps, there are plenty of stimulating outdoor activities, including mountain climbing, hiking, bungee jumping, hang gliding, fishing, skiing and snowboarding.

THAILAND

The Banyan Tree
33 Moo 4 Srisoonthorn Road
Cherngtalay
Amphur Talang
Phuket 83110
Thailand
Tel: +66 76 324374
Fax: +66 76 324375
E-mail: phuket@banyantree.com
With its blissful menu of treatments including the Oasis of Bliss and Voyage of Peace, the Banyan Tree Spa offers a deep sense of peace with deluxe pampering. Private Pool Villas ensure that you can have treatments in the most peaceful environment, undisturbed by your fellow guests.

Chiva-Som International Health Resort
73/4 Petchkasem Road
Hua Hin 77110
Thailand
Tel: +66 32 536536
Fax: +66 32 511154
With its beautiful pavilions and colonial-style apartments situated on 7 acres of pure white sandy beach, Chiva-Som offers a luxurious package of pampering and fitness, with a range of activities from aerobics, t'ai chi, yoga and meditation to healthy cookery classes, stress management and nutrition counselling. Relax in the flotation tank, partake of some sunset t'ai chi on the beach, be scrubbed, wrapped and pummelled or get super fit in the high-tech gym. Whatever you choose to do, rest assured that you will leave feeling and looking fitter and more relaxed.

The Oriental Spa at The Oriental Bangkok
48 Oriental Avenue
Bangkok 10500
Thailand
Tel: +66 22 360400/ 66 24 397613
Fax: +66 24 397587
The offspring of the historic hotel preferred by legendary writers such as Joseph Conrad, Somerset Maugham, James Michener and Noel Coward, this urban retreat with its dark wood interior and tropical treatments will leave you feeling calm and serene, not to mention utterly indulged. Set apart from the main hotel, the spa is reached by boat, giving it a unique feel of its own, while still reflecting the luxury of The Oriental.

UNITED KINGDOM

Agua at Sanderson
50 Berners Street
London W1P 3AD
UK
Tel: +44 (0)20 7300 1414
Fax: +44 (0)20 7300 1415
The sister spa of Agua at Delano in Miami, London's newest urban retreat is already attracting its fair share of attention. With its heavenly interior, designed by Philippe Starck, this Zen-like retreat in the heart of Ian Shrager's newest hotel offers a deluxe menu of treatments. Choose from massage, from Indian head massage to reiki; sumptuous body treatments, including the legendary Agua Milk and Honey and an ayurvedic-style massage with warm honey, sesame oil and milk. A selection of hydrotherapy treatments are available, including Swiss shower and underwater massage

Champneys at Tring
WiggingtonTring
Hertfordshire HP23 6HY
UK
Tel: +44 (0)1441 863351
Fax: +44 (0)1442 872342
Champneys has long been considered one of the most sumptuous spas in the UK with a luxurious Japanese-style treatment centre at its heart, luxurious accommodation and world class cuisine. Facilities include a spacious indoor pool and a fully equipped state-of-the-art gym, and the extensive range of fitness and relaxation classes, guided country hikes and beauty treatments ensure that mind, body and spirit will all be catered for.

The Cowshed at Babington House
Babington
Nr Frome
Somerset BA11 3RW
UK
Tel: +44 (0)1373 813860
E-mail: babingtonhouse@babhouse.co.uk
The Cowshed Spa is a jewel of a spa. With only four treatment rooms, it has a truly cosy and unique atmosphere, all within the luxurious grounds of Babington House, a modern country club with urban chic. Along with two heated pools, one indoor and one outdoor, a steam room, sauna and a compact high-tech gym, The Cowshed makes you feel special without any pretension. What really sets it apart, is the unique range of treatments including Cowgirl facial, using natural clay and essential oils, and the excellent Raw Hide body polish treatment. Accommodation comprises huge marshmallow-soft beds, freestanding bath tubs and enormous shower rooms. The food is utterly delicious – once you've checked in, you'll want to stay forever.

Forest Mere Health Farm
Liphook
Hampshire
GU30 7JQ
UK
Tel: +44 (0)1428 726000
Fax: +44 (0)1428 723501
Website: www.forestmere.co.uk
From thalassotherapy to Thai massage, Forest Mere offers a huge spa treatment menu for face and body in luxurious surroundings. For fitness addicts, there's everything from yoga and Pilates to t'ai chi and power walking together with all the latest fitness equipment and two swimming pools.

Henlow Grange Health Farm
Henlow
Bedfordshire SG16 6DB
UK
Tel: +44 (0)1462 811 111
Fax: +44 (0)1462 815 310
Website: www.henlowgrange.co.uk
One of the UK's best-loved health farms, Henlow Grange lies in 100 acres of unspoiled parkland and offers a range of accommodation from deluxe suites to modest standard rooms. Henlow is renowned for its fitness facilities, with many professional athletes coming here to train and unwind. A super-spacious swimming pool, state-of-the-art gymnasium and a mind-boggling selection

of fitness classes from aqua aerobics and step to dance and body conditioning. A wide variety of beauty treatments are also on offer at the spa's beauty centre, with reflexology, hydrotherapy and thalassotherapy-style baths and wraps. A delicious, nutritionally-balanced and calorie-counted menu ensures health-conscious eating

Hoar Cross Hall
Hoar Cross
Near Yoxall
Staffordshire DE13 8QS
UK
Tel: +44 (0)1283 575671
E-mail: info@hoarcross.co.uk
Websites:www.hoarcross.co.uk/
www.europeanayurveda.com
Hoar Cross Hall is one of England's most elegant stately home spa retreats. With luxurious surroundings it has a state-of-the-art spa with hydrotherapy baths, blitz jet showers, flotation therapy, saunas, steam rooms, water massage areas and a hydrotherapy pool. The hall also houses European Ayur-Veda Ltd, who provide a full range of stress-relieving ayurvedic therapies within a luxurious environment. Fitness activities include a full range of aerobics and body conditioning classes, yoga and meditation, tennis, cycling, golf, hiking, and swimming.

Lucknam Park
Colerne
Nr Bath
Wiltshire
SN14 8AZ
UK
Tel: +44 (0)1225 742777
Fax: +44 (0)1225 743536
Website: www.lucknampark.co.uk
Lucknam Park has one of the finest leisure spas in the country offering health, beauty and relaxation. The spa has an indoor swimming pool with doors opening on to sunny terraces and a traditional walled garden filled with roses. There is also a whirlpool spa, sauna, steam room, solarium and gym. A short distance from the spa is an entire house dedicated to massage and beauty treatments for men and women. The spa has been consistently voted as one of the top spas in the country by Condé Nast Traveller magazine readers.

Ragdale Hall Health Hydro
Ragdale Village
Nr Melton Mowbray
Leicestershire LE14 3PB
UK
Tel: +44 (0)1664 434831
Fax: +44 (0)1664 434587
E-mail: ragdalehall@btconnect.com
Website: www.ragdalehall.co.uk
Winner of the prestigious Health Spa of the Year award in 1999, Ragdale Hall is set in its own sprawling landscaped gardens in the Leicestershire countryside. With a comprehensive range of traditional and natural beauty therapies from deluxe facials and aromatherapy to detox treatments, Thai and shiatsu massage, reiki and Indian head massage, Ragdale is a truly holistic spa. To treat the mind, stress counselling, neuro linguistic programming, hypnotherapy and personal visualisation are available too, ensuring that every part of you is attended to. Alongside the usual fitness activities, such as aerobics, yoga, swimming and weight training, you can try your hand at archery, fencing and lazer shooting. And to satisfy your appetite, Ragdale's menu is a combination of healthy, delicious and beautifully presented foods.

St David's Hotel and Spa
Havannah Street
Cardiff Bay
Cardiff CF10 5SD
UK
Tel: +44 (0)2920 313084
Fax: +44 (0)2920 487056
E-mail: reservations@fivestar-htl-wales.com
Website: www.rfhotels.com
This newly built five-star hotel overlooking Cardiff Bay houses the equally beautiful St David's Spa. State-of-the-art architecture fuses with world class service and the ultimate in modern luxury. A hydrotherapy spa with seaweed, salt and trace minerals helps to rejuvenate, while a full range of beauty treatments using E'Spa products leave you feeling relaxed and de-stressed. A fully equipped gym, exercise pool and two marine hydro pools complete the spa experience and a spa dining area provides healthy haute cuisine.

Stobo Castle Health Spa
Stobo
Peeblesshire
Scotland EH45 8NY
UK
Tel: +44 (0)1721 760249
Fax: +44 (0)1721 760294
Situated in the midst of a stunning Scottish landscape, Stobo Castle manages to combine old-style charm with modern luxury. With a relaxed country house party-style atmosphere, delicious low-fat, health conscious menu and the incredibly luxurious spa with under-floor heating, Stobo offers an all-round spa experience that can be tailor-made to the individual. From pampering facials and body treatments to an array of indoor and outdoor fitness activities, you will leave Stobo feeling totally rejuvenated.

UNITED STATES OF AMERICA

Agua at Delano
1685 Collins Avenue
Miami Beach
Florida FL 33139
USA
Tel: +1 305 672 2000
Fax: +1 305 532 0099
Agua has to be the hippest health spa in the universe, not least because it is perched on top of the fabulously cool Delano Hotel. The bathhouse overlooks the Atlantic Ocean and is decorated in the same heavenly, serene style as the main hotel, complete with billowy white curtains and comfy daybeds. Try the delicious milk and honey treatment based on an ancient ayurvedic recipe, wallow in the huge spa baths and enjoy every kind of massage imaginable. No wonder it's Madonna's favourite.

The Ashram
2025 North McKain Street
Calabasas
California
USA
Tel: +1 818 222 6900
Don't expect luxury at this glorified 'boot camp', but do expect to leave, fitter and firmer. A favourite with Cindy Crawford, Ashley Judd and Oprah Winfrey, The Ashram offers a strict programme of low-calorie vegetarian food, daily mountain hikes, yoga and meditation – and if you're really lucky, an end-of-the-day massage to undo all the knots and melt away muscle aches and pains.

Cal-A-Vie
San Diego
California
USA
Tel: +1 760 945 2055
Fax: +1 760 630 0074

Built in the style of a Provencal village, Cal-A-Vie is a deluxe retreat with just 24 private cottages. With a devoted clientele, including Kathleen Turner, a week at Cal-A-Vie costs around $5000. The package includes all meals, spa treatments, aerobics, hiking, water exercises, yoga, tai chi, weight training and stretch classes. Expensive but worth it.

Canyon Ranch Health Resort

8600 East Rockcliff Road
Tucson
Arizona 85750
USA
Tel: +1 520 749 9000
Fax: +1 520 749 1646
Website: www.canyonranch.com
Deservedly winner of many top international spa awards, Canyon Ranch is one of the most inspiring retreats in the world. Set in the foothills of the Santa Catalina Mountains, the Ranch sits in 70 acres of stunning Sonoran Desert. One of the fundamental aims of the spa is not just to pamper you and get you fit, but to teach you how to adapt what you learn at the spa and take it home with you. Enjoy a huge range of bodywork treatments from ayurvedic shirodhara, where warm oil is slowly dripped on face and body, to canyon stone massage, where smooth basalt rocks are used to release tension throughout your body and any number of facials. Fitness activities, including desert hikes, cycling, racquet sports and golf, are topped off by the delicious world-renowned Canyon Ranch cuisine.

Eden Roc Resort and Spa

4525 Collins Avenue
Miami Beach
Florida 33140
USA
Tel. +1 305 674 5585
Website: www.edenrocresort.com
This Art Deco masterpiece houses the luxurious Spa of Eden with its huge array of fitness activities including aerobics, yoga, ballet, box aerobics, step, slide, boating, swimming, tennis and squash and beauty treats such as reflexology, shiatsu massage, body wraps and every facial imaginable. The spa cuisine is both healthy and appealing with influences from around the world.

The Expanding Light

Nevada City
California
USA
Tel: +1 530 478 7518

Yoga and meditation are the focus at The Expanding Light, a simple but beautiful spa where private rooms are offered alongside dormitory-style accommodation – not everyone's cup of tea. Delicious vegetarian cuisine is the perfect accompaniment to the holistic therapies and activities at The Expanding Light, but the yoga classes are probably what brings people back, time and time again. Depending on the season, cross-country and downhill skiing are also available.

Golden Door

PO Box 463077
Escondido
California 92046 3077
USA
Tel: +1 760 744 6677
Fax: +1 760 591 3048
One of my own personal favourites, the Golden Door has an Eastern feel, with its Zen-style landscaped gardens, ornamental Carp ponds and Japanese-inspired architecture. Brilliant for both fitness and relaxation, take advantage of the morning mountain hike, the extensive yoga and meditation and the gorgeous Japanese bathhouse, where you can wallow in the evening before hitting the sack. The food at the Golden Door is also unmissable, the perfect combination of healthy and delicious.

Green Valley Fitness Resort and Spa

Utah
USA
Tel: +1 435 628 8060
Fax: +1 435 673 4084
At the Green Valley Spa, the day starts with a two-hour morning hike through Zion National Park with stunning red rock canyon scenery. The spa itself is an adobe-style village with a huge selection of fitness and beauty facilities including professional tennis coaching, a mind and body centre for stress reduction and a luxurious spa treatment centre offering everything from aromatic water treatments and massages to pedicures and reflexology.

The Greenhouse

PO Box 1144
Arlington
Texas 76004 1144
USA
Tel: +1 817 640 4000
Website: www.thegreenhousespa.com
Exclusively for women, The Greenhouse is an incredibly luxurious spa offering a huge array of activities and pampering treatments in a

tranquil and charming environment, reminiscent of a colonial mansion. Privacy and individual service is the order of the day, with breakfast being delivered to your room every morning, along with your personalized daily schedule. Fitness activities on offer include tae bo and Pilates and the spa includes Vichy, Swiss and Scotch Hose showers.

Lake Austin Spa Resort

1705 South Quinlan Park Road
Austin
Texas 78732
USA
Tel: +1 512 372 7300
Fax: +1 512 266 1572
Website: www.lakeaustin.com
An oasis of calm on the shores of Lake Austin, here the emphasis is on stress reduction, inner strength and top-to-toe holistic revitalisation. From t'ai chi to kayaking, there are a huge number of activities designed to induce relaxation and to boost all-round fitness levels. The food is wholesome and mainly organic and the beauty treatments on offer are a combination of homemade treatments, such as the honey mango scrub. Very low key and very chilled out.

The Lodge at Skylonda

16350 Skyline Blvd
Woodside
California 94062
USA
Tel: +1 650 851 6625
Fax: +1 650 851 5504
E-mail: info@skylondalodge.com
Website: www.skylondalodge.com
Resting in the redwood forests of northern California, The Lodge at Skylonda is a restful, private retreat with a deluxe spa programme. With this a prime location for hiking, guides will take you through the majestic forests along a variety of trails that cater for both the beginner and the expert. A fully equipped state-of-the-art gym, indoor pool, yoga and aerobics programme means that there is something for everyone, together with an excellent pampering menu. The Lodge is also famed for its low-fat cuisine with a delicious repertoire of seafood, roasts and ragouts.

Ojai Valley Inn and Spa

Country Club Road
Ojai
California 93023
USA
Tel: +1 805 646 1111

Located in the Ojai valley, an area of great natural beauty with the Topa Topa Mountains as a backdrop, this Spanish village-style spa is the perfect escape if you long for a taste of the outdoors together with the ultimate in pampering. The Spa Ojai has an art studio, meditation gardens, outdoor fireplaces and a Chumash Indian interpretative trail, together with 28 treatment rooms, many of which have their own fireplaces. For the active, there's a choice of riding, cycling, boating and hiking plus a wide selection of yoga, t'ai chi and a unique yoga and bodywork-based exercise regime. Renowned for their Kuyam mud treatment and Petals bath, the Ojai beauty rooms are well worth checking out.

The Palms at Palm Springs
572 N. Indian Canyon Drive
Palm Springs
California 92262
USA
Tel: +1 760 325 1111
Full ranges of activities are available at a reasonable cost at The Palms, including aerobics, yoga, meditation, hiking, golf, riding, beauty treatments and massage. The Spanish-style setting and spacious rooms ensure a restful stay while the low-calorie and low-cholesterol menu adds up to a super-healthy but delicious diet.

Professional Golfers Association of America Resort and Spa
400 Avenue of the Champions
Palm Beach Gardens
Florida 33418
USA
Tel: +1 561 624 8400
With its six stunning 'waters of the world' outdoor therapy pools, featuring mineral salts from the Dead Sea and the Pyrenées and 31 treatment rooms, The PGA resort offers world class spa and sports facilities. The resort also offers a five-tournament golf course, a seven-mile hiking trail, 19 tennis courts and a huge indoor fitness centre with all the latest equipment.

The Spa Grande at the Grand Wailea Resort
Maui
Hawaii
USA
Tel: +1 808 875 1234
If luxury and indulgence are high on your list of priorities, The Spa Grande will suit you down to the ground. Every room at the hotel has a beautiful sea view, while the spa's

speciality is hydrotherapy featuring Japanese-style baths, loofah scrubs, a Roman plunge tub and speciality baths including papaya enzyme, seaweed, mineral salt and aromatherapy. Fitness activities include aerobics, yoga, hiking, cycling. water sports and weight training. For those with children, the hotel provides fantastic recreational facilities including a day camp, cinema and outdoor pool, allowing parents to chill out at the spa while the children are entertained.

Ten Thousand Waves
PO Box 10200
Santa Fe
New Mexico 87504
USA
Tel: +1 505 992 5025
Fax: +1 505 989 5077
Ten Thousand Waves combines the best of Santa Fe style with a traditional Japanese spa. Perched up in the hills above Santa Fe, the spa nestles among pinon pines and cedar trees. Treatments centre on the individual and communal hot tubs where you can happily wallow for hours undisturbed, just enjoying the scenery and the bubbling waters. Treatments are of the highest standard and you'll find unusual massages such as watsu, where you are cradled in the water by a therapist and Japanese hot stone massage, where basalt and marble stones are heated with warm oils and used to massage your whole body. The spa is open as a day resort or you can stay in one of the eight Houses of the Moon, luxurious Japanese guest suites.

Two Bunch Palms
Desert Hot Springs
California
USA
Tel: +1 760 329 8791
Once the bolt hole of Al Capone, Two Bunch Palms is now one of America's best-loved luxury spa destinations. Set in a lush oasis of palm trees, tamarisks and bougainvillaea, the spa is famed for its sensual body massages, mud baths, mineral hot springs and body wraps. Fitness facilities are also available and the Living Essence Cuisine ensures that a healthy diet is followed.

Vista Clara Ranch Health Spa
Galisteo
New Mexico
USA
Tel: +1 505 466 4772
E-mail: vclara@newmexico.com
Website: www.vistaclara.com

Situated in the awe-inspiring setting of the New Mexico plains with its terracotta cliffs and pinon-studded canyons, the hacienda-style adobe buildings of Vista Clara fit in perfectly with the landscape and the Native American theme carries through the spa. A ceremonial kiva is used for fitness and dance classes, there's an authentic tepee and sweat lodge on the grounds and treatments using ingredients local to the area are incorporated into the spa's treatment menu. The food is an absolutely delicious, health-conscious gourmet menu, with my own personal favourite being the sumptuous breakfasts with homemade oatmeal, muffins, fresh fruit and home-baked breads. Vista Clara also has all the latest fitness equipment, an ozone pool and Jacuzzi and fantastic cross-country hikes guaranteed to chase away the cobwebs and awaken every underused muscle.

Westward Look Resort
245 East Ina Road
Tucson
Arizona 85704
USA
Tel: +1 520 297 1151
Fax: +1 520 297 9023
Website: www.westwardlook.com
Nestled in the foothills above Tucson, Arizona, Westward Look is an 80-acre ranch-style resort which boasts a world class tennis centre, a fitness trail, riding, yoga and meditation to name but a few of the activities on its menu. The food is a mix of Native American, Spanish and Arizona-Anglo cooking, together with the health-conscious Catalina Cuisine menu. The treatments are bliss.

The Wyndham Resort and Spa (formerly The Bonaventure)
250 Racquet Club Road
Fort Lauderdale
33326 Florida
USA
Tel: +1 954 389 3300
Fax: +1 954 384 1416
Website: www.wyndham.com
Renowned for its sports facilities, The Wyndham will appeal to those after a seriously active spa holiday. From two championship golf courses, six tennis courts, and five outdoor swimming pools to a roller skating rink, a bowling alley and an array of boating activities, there is an endless menu of physical pursuits. Relaxation is guaranteed at the treatment spa offering array hydrotherapy treats and face and body pampering.

SPA	Most tranquil	Best for fitness	Alternative treatments	Plush pampering	Best food	Price
AUSTRALIA						
Azabu	★		★	★		Deluxe
The Cape Retreat		★		★		Moderate
Couran Cove Resort Spa and Total Living Centre		★				Moderate
Daintree Eco-Lodge and Spa	★		★		★	Moderate
Eaglereach Wilderness Resort		★				Moderate
Empire Retreat	★	★		★		Moderate
The Golden Door Health Retreat	★			★	★	Deluxe
Hyatt Regency-Coolum		★		★	★	Moderate
The Observatory Hotel Spa	★	★			★	Deluxe
The Sanctuary Holistic Retreat	★	★	★	★		Budget
Shizuka Ryokan	★					Deluxe
Solar Springs Health Retreat	★	★				Moderate
CANADA						
Echo Valley Ranch Resort	★	★		★		Moderate
Mountain Trek Fitness Retreat and Health Spa		★	★			Budget
Solace Spa at Banff Springs Hotel	★	★		★	★	Deluxe
THE CARIBBEAN						
La Casa de Vida Natural	★		★	★		Budget
Le Sport	★	★		★		Deluxe
FRANCE						
Caudalie Institut de Vinotherapie	★			★		Moderate
Domaine du Royal Club Evian	★	★		★	★	Deluxe
Institute of Thalassatherapy Louison Bobet	★	★		★		Moderate
GERMANY						
Brenner's Park Hotel	★	★		★		Deluxe
INDIA						
The Kairali Ayurvedic Health Resort	★		★			Moderate
The Spa at Rajvilas	★		★	★	★	Deluxe
The Taj Ayurvedic Centre	★		★			Moderate
INDONESIA						
The Banyan Tree, Bintan	★	★		★	★	Deluxe
Jamu Traditional Spa	★		★	★		Budget
The Jimbaran Spa at The Four Seasons Resort	★		★	★		Deluxe
The Mandara Spa at The Chedi	★		★	★		Deluxe
The Mandara Spa at The Ibah	★			★		Deluxe
Nusa Dua Beach Hotel and Spa	★			★	★	Deluxe
The Oberoi, Bali	★		★	★	★	Deluxe
The Oberoi, Lombok	★		★	★	★	Deluxe
Spa at The Bali Hyatt	★			★		Deluxe
ISRAEL						
Carmel Forest Spa Resort	★	★	★	★		Moderate
Radisson Moriah Plaza Dead Sea Spa Hotel			★	★		Moderate
ITALY						
Palazzo Arzaga Spa	★			★	★	Deluxe

It's not just activities and services that are important, a spa break also needs to be tailored to your budget. So we've given a rough guide to pricing in the following categories, based on a week's stay:
• Budget – £800 or under   • Moderate – £800 to £1500   • Deluxe – £1500 and upwards.

SPA	Most tranquil	Best for fitness	Alternative treatments	Plush pampering	Best food	Price
MALAYSIA						
The Mandara Spa at The Datai	★				★	Deluxe
MEXICO						
Punta Serena	★		★			Budget
Rancho La Puerta	★	★	★		★	Moderate
The Spa at Las Ventanas al Paradiso	★		★	★	★	Deluxe
SWITZERLAND						
The Grand Hotel and Spa Victoria-Jungfrau	★	★		★	★	Moderate
THAILAND						
The Banyan Tree, Phuket						Deluxe
Chiva-Som International Health Resort	★		★	★		Deluxe
The Oriental Spa at The Oriental Bangkok	★	★			★	Deluxe
UNITED KINGDOM				★	★	
Agua at Sanderson						Deluxe
Champneys at Tring	★					Deluxe
The Cowshed at Babington House	★	★	★			Deluxe
Forest Mere Health Farm	★	★	★			Moderate
Henlow Grange Health Farm		★		★	★	Moderate
Hoar Cross Hall		★		★	★	Moderate
Lucknam Park		★			★	Moderate
Ragdale Hall Health Hydro	★			★	★	Moderate
St David's Hotel and Spa		★	★	★		Moderate
Stobo Castle Health Spa		★		★	★	Deluxe
UNITED STATES OF AMERICA	★	★				
Agua at Delano						Deluxe
The Ashram	★	★		★	★	Deluxe
Cal-A-Vie		★				Deluxe
Canyon Ranch Health Resort	★	★		★	★	Moderate
Eden Roc Resort and Spa	★	★	★	★	★	Deluxe
The Expanding Light	★		★	★	★	Budget
Golden Door	★	★	★			Deluxe
Green Valley Fitness Resort and Spa	★	★		★	★	Moderate
The Greenhouse	★	★				Deluxe
Lake Austin Spa Resort	★	★		★	★	Moderate
The Lodge at Skylonda	★	★		★	★	Moderate
Ojai Valley Inn and Spa		★	★	★		Moderate
The Palms at Palm Springs	★	★	★	★		Moderate
Professional Golfers Association of America Resort and Spa		★		★		Deluxe / Deluxe
The Spa Grande at the Grand Wailea Resort		★		★	★	Moderate
Ten Thousand Waves	★			★		Deluxe
Two Bunch Palms	★			★	★	Moderate
Vista Clara Ranch Health Spa	★	★	★			Moderate
Westward Look Resort	★	★	★	★	★	Moderate
The Wyndham Resort and Spa		★		★		

However, almost every spa we've mentioned does a huge variety of packages including two and three night stays, mid-week breaks and so on, to suit all budgets and time requirements.

Home-spa suppliers

BATHROOM ACCESSORIES

Czech & Speake
Tel: +44 (0)800 919728
Exquisite bathroom fixtures and fittings, plus beautiful range of bath and body products, deluxe scented candles and burning sticks.

Fired Earth H20 Bathrooms
Tel: +44 (0)1295 812088
Beautiful sinks, baths, towel rails, tiles, fixtures and fittings.

Habitat
Tel: +44 (0)845 6010740 for nearest branch
Pared down bathroom fittings including towel rails, mirrors, soap dishes and storage containers.

CP Hart
Tel: +44 (0)20 7902 1000
One of the largest stockists of designer bathroom wares, including spa baths and whirlpools, state-of-the-art showers and beautiful fittings.

Aston Matthews
Tel: +44 (0)20 7226 7220
Huge range of bathroom fixtures and fittings, baths, sinks, hot tubs and showers.

Mira
Tel: +44 (0)870 8400035
For the best power showers.

Original Bathrooms
Tel: +44 (0)20 8940 7554
Innovative bathroom suppliers stocking exclusive designs in stainless steel. Spa-style bath and body products

Acqua di Parma
Tel: +44 (0)20 7328 1036 for stockists
Beautiful Italian-made soaps, colognes, scented candles, bath and body creams, powders and lotions.

Aromatherapy Associates
Tel: +44 (0)20 7371 9878
High quality aromatherapy oils, massage and bath preparations.

Aveda
Tel: +44 (0)20 7410 1600 for stockists
Cult beauty products inspired by ancient ayurvedic know-how, including body cleansers, skin creams and toners and scented candles.

Bach Flower Remedies
Tel: +44 (0)20 7495 2404
Cult flower remedies including the acclaimed Rescue Remedy, useful for treating emotional ailments.

Bath and Body Works
Tel: +44 (0)20 7580 0707 for stockists
Fantastic selection of body scrubs, scented candles, bath treats and accessories at budget prices.

Borghese
Tel: +44 (0)1273 408800 for stockists
Famous for therapeutic spa-style mineral muds, body scrubs and mineral enriched face and body preparations originating from the renowned Montecatini region of Italy.

Cariad
Tel: +44 (0)1932 269921 for stockists
High quality aromatherapy bath and body preparations and essential oils.

Caudalie
Tel: +44 (0)1202 890339
Grape-based skin preparations for bath, body and face from the French 'Grape Vine' Spa.

Crabtree & Evelyn
Tel: +44 (0)20 7603 1611
Purveyors of spa-style face and body products, scented candles and aromatherapy-based preparations.

Elemis
Tel: +44 (0)20 8954 8033
Premium quality, plant-based face and body preparations used at over 300 spas internationally.

E'Spa
Tel: +44 (0)1252 741600 for stockists
Used in some of the world's most exclusive spas, the E'Spa range includes soothing skin treatments, seaweed enriched bath preparations and aromatherapy-based bath and body oils.

L'Occitane
Tel: +44 (0)20 7290 1420
For delicious aromatherapy oils, foam baths, bath salts, candles, body brushes and soaps.

Neal's Yard Remedies
Tel: +44 (0)20 7627 1949 for stockists
Wonderful array of aromatherapy-based oils, bath, body and skin products and bath accessories including body brushes and mitts.

Origins
Tel: + 44 (0)800 731 4039 for stockists
Face and body products chock-full with naturally derived skin-enhancing ingredients, including the legendary Salt Rub body scrub, Liquid Clay foaming cleanser and Soothing Sea Salts for the bath. Brilliant selection of body brushes and bath mitts.

Repecharge
Tel: +44 (0)800 7317546 for details
Luxurious seaweed and mineral-based spa skin bath and body products including body creams and restorative bath preparations.

Space NK
Tel: +44 (0)20 7299 4999
A treasure trove of spa-style products from companies such as E'Spa, Philosophy, Remede, Nuxe, Kiehl's and own-line Space NK bath and body, including scented candles, foam baths and incense sticks.

Further reading

Tisserand
Tel: +44 (0)1273 325666 for stockists
Excellent quality essential oils and aromatherapy-based products.

Virgin Vie
Tel: +44 (0)870 9099095 for stockists
Wide range of affordable spa-inspired bath and body products, including the Spa Treat range.

DIRECT FROM THE SPA ...

Experience a taste of the spa lifestyle with the following home-spa products.

Mandara Spa
Tel: +62 361 755 575 or e-mail
jmatthews@mandaraspa.com
Beautiful range of Mandara Massage Oils, soaps, bath and body products.

Nusa Dua Beach Hotel and Spa
Tel: +62 361 771210 or
e-mail ndbhnet@indosat.net.id.
The Esens range of spa products created by spa consultants, Kim and Cary Collier, includes a DIY Lalur Kit, one-shot massage oils and luxurious bath preparations. Also available direct from Esens, tel: +62 361 771 991 or e-mail Collierspas@hotmail.com.

Westward Look Resort
Tel: +1 520 297 0134 or check out www.westwardlook.com for further details
Try The Revitalizer Kit, including a Westward Look robe, Sensi massage sandals, Stress Relief Bath Therapy Kit including massage and body oil, bath salts and natural sea sponge. A wide selection of herbal and bath teas are also available.

BATHROOMS

Bathroom by Suzanne Ardley (Dorling Kindersley)
Colours of the Soul by June McLeod (Piatkus)
Colour Healing Manual by Pauline Willis (Piatkus)
Essence of White by Hilary Mandleberg (Ryland, Peters & Small)
Pure Style by Jane Cumberbatch (Ryland, Peters & Small)
The Sensual Home by Ilse Crawford (Quadrille)

RELAXATION

The Bloomsbury Encyclopaedia of Aromatherapy by Chrissie Wildwood (Bloomsbury)
The Complete Illustrated Guide to Yoga by Howard Kent (Element)
Lazy Person's Guide to Emotional Healing by Andrew Tresidder (Newleaf)
Natural Healing by Chrissie Wildwood (Piatkus)
The New Book of Yoga by Lucy Liddell (Ebury Press)
Tree of Yoga by B.K.S. Iyengar (Aquarian Press)

SPA FOOD

Canyon Ranch Cooking – Bringing the Spa Home by Jeanne Jones (Harper Collins)
Champneys Cookbook – 100 Innovative Recipes for Healthy Eating by Adam Palmer (Ward Lock)
The Golden Door Cookbook by Michel Stroot (Broadway)
Great Tastes – Healthy Cooking From Canyon Ranch (Canyon Ranch)
The Rancho La Puerta Cookbook by Bill Wavrin (Broadway)

FACE AND BODY TREATS

The Book of Ayurveda by Judith H. Morrison (Gaia Books)
Indian Beauty Secrets by Monisha Bharadwaj (Kyle Cathie)
Marie Claire Style, Bathing by Jane Campsie (Murdoch Books)
The Tropical Spa by Sophie Benge (Periplus)

Index

Acknowledgements

A massive thank you to the following for their contributions to this project.

Researcher Kate Hames for all her hard work, faxing, e-mailing and phone calling around the globe.

My best-mate-down-under, Melinda Aldridge for all her assistance and persistence on the Aussie front.

And the following photographers: Brian Nice, for his beautiful and inspiring images, endless Fed Ex packages and transatlantic support; Simon Brown, for allowing us to use his gorgeous bathroom and bathing pictures; Stefano Massimo for permitting us to use some of his wonderful photographs.

Denise Bates, for her constant support, endless patience and serenity – even when the going was tough!

Emma Callery, for her attention to detail, wonderful editing and overall loveliness throughout.

Ciara Lunn, for keeping up with it all and tracking me down when needed!

Helen Lewis, for her inspirational design.

Carol Pullen, for the inspiration, endless cups of Rosie Lee and for keeping me motivated when my energy was flagging.

Sue, Hazel and Frances Sherar, for all the moral support and encouragement, not to mention the long walks!

Thanks to all at New Romney Junior and Infants Schools for their constant support, especially Michele Rowland, Mrs Brown, Mrs Haldane and all their pupils.

Huge thanks also goes to the following people for their help, contributions, recipes, and shared secrets! Belinda Shepherd at The Four Seasons; Sue Arnett in the public relations department for Rancho La Puerta and Golden Door; Katie Garber at Canyon Ranch; Mary Beth Chambers at Lake Austin Spa Resort; Marilyn Carr at The Expanding Light; Donna Kreutz at the Westward Look Resort; Merrill Williams at Ojai Valley Inn and Spa; Annie Kinnane at the Couran Cove Resort; Norman Dove at Echo Valley Ranch Resort, Canada; Clare and Caroline at Ann Scott Associates, London; Clare Branch at St David's Hotel & Spa; Anne Hart at Henlow Grange; Gillie Turner at Champneys; Angela Hopkins at the Hyatt Regency Coolum; Belinda Anderson at The Golden Door Health Retreat, Australia; Veda Dante at Daintree Eco Lodge & Spa; Vicki Taylor at Ragdale Hall; fitness expert Dean Hodgkin; Mr Yasin Zargar at Indus Tours and Travel Ltd; John Wallwork and Michael Jacques at T'ai Chi UK, tel: 020 7407 4775 or visit the website at www.taichiuk.co.uk; Sean Harrington from Elemis; Sue Harmsworth from E'Spa; Leila Fazel at Agua; Lydia Sarfati at Repechage.

The copyright for the Native Body Glow recipe on page 86 rests with Vista Clara Ranch Health Spa.

The publishers thank the following photographers and organisations for the photographs that appear in this book

Page 1 Stefano Massimo, 2 Brian Nice, 4 top Brian Nice, 4 bottom Craig Robertson, 7 Brian Nice, 8 Arcaid (Richard Powers), 10 Simon Brown, 13 Simon Brown, 17 x 4 Simon Brown, 20 Simon Brown, 24 Brian Nice, 29 Brian Nice, 33 Tony Stone Images (Andrea Booher), 36 x 4 Retna (Philip Reeson), 44 Craig Robertson, 49 Craig Robertson, 56 Craig Robertson, 61 Craig Robertson, 64 Craig Robertson, 68 Stefano Massimo, 71 Brian Nice, 72 Brian Nice, 75 top left Tony Stone Images (Laurent Monneret), 75 top right, bottom left and right Brian Nice, 76 Brian Nice, 84 Brian Nice, 89 x 4 Simon Brown, 93 Brian Nice, 97 Brian Nice, 98 Brian Nice, 101 x 4 Simon Brown, 104 Brian Nice, 109 Brian Nice, 111 Brian Nice, 112 top left and right, bottom right Simon Brown, 112 bottom left PWA, 116 Brian Nice, 121 Brian Nice, 125 Stefano Massimo, 128 Stefano Massimo.

All illustrations by Lynne Robinson